COMMUNICATING CARE AT THE END OF LIFE

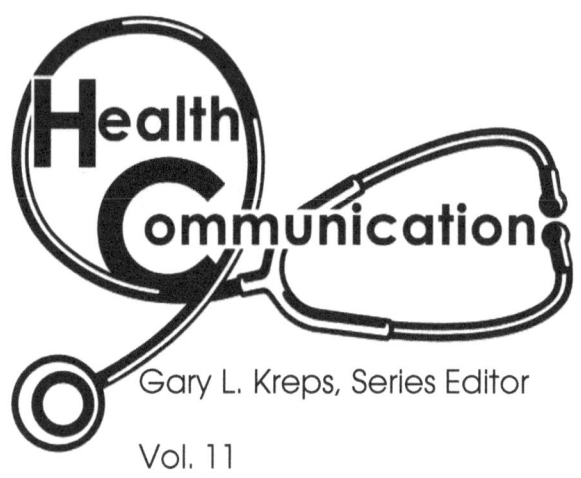

Health Communication

Gary L. Kreps, Series Editor

Vol. 11

The Health Communication series is part of
the Peter Lang Media and Communication list.
Every volume is peer reviewed and meets
the highest quality standards for content and production.

PETER LANG
New York • Bern • Frankfurt • Berlin
Brussels • Vienna • Oxford • Warsaw

CAREY CANDRIAN

COMMUNICATING CARE AT THE END OF LIFE

PETER LANG
New York • Bern • Frankfurt • Berlin
Brussels • Vienna • Oxford • Warsaw

Library of Congress Cataloging-in-Publication Data
Candrian, Carey, author.
Communicating care at the end of life / Carey Candrian.
p. cm. — (Health communication; vol. 11)
Includes bibliographical references and index.
1. Terminal care—psychology. 2. Attitude to death.
3. Communication. 4. Death. I. Title.
II. Series: Health communication (New York, N.Y.); v. 11.
R726.8   362.17'5—dc23   2014024784
ISBN 978-1-4331-2714-4 (hardcover)
ISBN 978-1-4539-1403-8 (e-book)
ISSN 2153-1277

Bibliographic information published by **Die Deutsche Nationalbibliothek**.
Die Deutsche Nationalbibliothek lists this publication in the "Deutsche
Nationalbibliografie"; detailed bibliographic data are available
on the Internet at http://dnb.d-nb.de/.

The paper in this book meets the guidelines for permanence and durability
of the Committee on Production Guidelines for Book Longevity
of the Council of Library Resources.

© 2015 Peter Lang Publishing, Inc., New York
29 Broadway, 18th floor, New York, NY 10006
www.peterlang.com

Printed in Germany

For everybody who loves
For everybody who suffers
For everybody who cares

CONTENTS

SERIES EDITOR'S PREFACE

Gary L. Kreps, Ph.D.

Communicating Care at the End of Life is a very personal and most revealing exploration of the communication dynamics that influence the dying process, based on the author's extensive personal experiences in both hospital emergency departments and in hospices. The author, Carey Candrian, explores what it takes to die well, to have a good death, examining the communication factors that lead to a comfortable, dignified, and satisfying death for all participants. She also analyzes the communication processes used to make sense of death. There are many lessons to be learned from this book that can help guide effective communication at the end of life.

The book raises a number of important and complex questions about how we can use strategic and sensitive communication to help demystify and soften the challenges experienced when working through the dying process. For example, what are the unique communication needs of individuals who are confronting the end of their lives? How can we help these individuals create a sense of meaning and control over this unfamiliar process of transitioning from living to dying. What can be done to support family members and friends as they prepare for the deaths of their loved ones? What can health care providers do to promote a good death, while meeting their own personal uncertainties and concerns about death and dying? How can we design health care systems, policies, practices, and communication technologies to support the key stakeholders during the dying process? Carey Candrian addresses these complex issues in this book by vividly recounting and analyzing rich and revealing stories about her own personal experiences observing and participating in the dying process, the experiences of many of her health care professional colleagues delivering care and support during clients' deaths, and the experiences of patients and their loved ones when confronting death. Many of these stories illustrate good communication strategies (best practices) for supporting the content and relational needs of those who are confronting death. While other stories provide more cautionary tales about how communication may not have been handled particularly well to promote a comfortable passing for all participants in the dying process. However, all of the stories invite the reader to vicariously experience the complex interpersonal dynamics of communicating to facilitate the best possible outcomes from death and dying.

I learned a great deal from this book that will help me prepare for my own death, the deaths of my loved ones, and will help me support the personal needs and concerns of others who are confronting death. Too often, particularly in the Western world, we avoid examining the dynamics of death and dying. It is too uncomfortable for many of us to examine and discuss these issues. However, this failure to examine the complexities of death and dying can leave us poorly prepared to respond when death comes to our door (and sooner or later it will come to your door). Death is an inevitable part of life, and we all need to develop the communication skills needed for making sense of mortality and supporting the information needs of our loved ones. If you are a health care provider (either a formal professional provider or an informal family caregiver), it is most likely that you will need to develop strategic communication skills for responding to the complexities of death and dying. This powerful and important book can help you address the complexities of the dying process and enable you to promote comfortable and satisfying transitions for all of the participants in the dying process.

ACKNOWLEDGMENTS

This project would not be without the help, guidance, and support of many. First, thank you to Stan Deetz. I could not have done any of this without you, your ideas and your support. Next, thank you to Mary Savigar, Sophie Appel, and Gary Kreps for your insightful and thoughtful review, and for being so delightful to work with. Thank you to Susan and Gerry for your incredible wisdom and help over the years, and for inviting me into the emergency department and hospice. And thank you to Jean Kutner for sharing your belief in palliative care and the relationship between communication and care with me a long time ago.

Thanks especially to the patients, families and health care workers I have shared moments, hours and days with who are not listed on this page but infuse every single one of the following pages. I have been humbled in many ways having met you all. And many of you have shown me—and some have made me feel—the difference between life and living, a lesson far more important than I could have learned on my own. Finally, thank you to my incredible family—Bev, Scott, Jeff, Jody and Ibby—for understanding, supporting and caring for me beyond words. And thank you to Leo, the love of my life, for being the way you are.

INTRODUCTION

"Do not ask me to remember, don't try to make me understand. Let me rest and know you're with me, kiss my cheek and hold my hand. I'm confused beyond your concept, I'm sad and sick and lost. All I know is that I need you, to be with me at all cost. Do not lose your patience with me, do not scold or curse or cry. I can't help the way I'm acting, I can't be different though I try. Just remember that I need you, that the best of me is gone. Please don't fail to stand beside me, love me 'til my life is gone.'"—Owen Darnell

Introduction

The aging of the population is one of the major public health challenges of the 21st century (Centers for Disease Control and Prevention, 2012). Additionally, the cost of providing care for an older person is three to five times greater than the cost of someone under 65. As a result, the demands for healthcare services for an aging population are exploding. Furthermore, the demand for these services across the world is increasing alongside an astonishing rate of medical error; devastating rates of loneliness among the elderly—a risk factor for early death comparable to smoking 15 cigarettes a day; the inability to follow patient preferences around the end of life; competing visions of how to best organize systems of care delivery for the elderly; and international reports of widespread stress, burnout, and compassion fatigue among those who care for the terminally ill. Consequently, health care needs are growing ever more complex, especially around the elderly, characterized by more to know, more to do, more to manage, more to organize, more to watch, more to feel, and more people involved than ever before.

I spent two years deeply engaged in two diverse settings: an emergency department (ED) and a hospice. I have worked ethnographically, capturing in detail the words and actions used in caring for seriously ill people. I understand ethnography to be a written means of representing and presenting a culture by describing and understanding localized practices, particularly communicative practices. Further, understanding these practices helps me to uncover how talk produces and reproduces certain meanings, norms, and strategies around the end of life. Even more, I believe that to do ethnography is to subject myself, my body, my personality, my social condition to the set of circumstances that play upon a group of individuals so that I am close to them as they are responding to what life does to them. Capturing the voices, the utterances, the pauses, and the hesitations in their unique formations is central to ethnography. Therefore, the quotes throughout this book have not been altered for the simple reason that something significant would be lost if the language were to be cleaned up. Entering health care settings, like hospice and the ED, is difficult because they are often filled with indelicate odors, sights, sounds, and because they are places where sick and not-so-sick bodies are overworked, overstressed, and underappreciated. They are also settings that cut to the core of who we are; what it means to be a patient; what it means to be a provider, and the role we must play and the skills we need to perfect that role. In essence, they pull and pound on our hearts and souls in the name of healing. And through their organization, these settings orient us to reflect on the meaning of life and the meaning of death in a particular way. What follows is a brief orientation to these settings, taken from my interactions with the sites.

Setting: Hospice of Saints (HOS)

Date: Tuesday, 28 April 2007, clock reads 15:30

Note to volunteers from the nursing station: *Sandra, who will be 68 in December and lost her eyesight two years ago, is feeling especially confused today about why she was admitted to hospice last week. Please help her process the transition. If she asks whether she is dying, do not try and respond immediately with words; listen patiently and empathetically.*

Setting: Sage Medical Center (SMC), Emergency Department

Date: Friday, 7 December 2008, clock reads 22:01

"Sad situation in bed one, I'll fill you in," Doc says. She pushes out a rolling swivel chair for me as she is looking at a recent patient chart. She mentions some medical terms and numbers, most of which are incomprehensible to me. She interrupts herself and says, "enough of this, let's go see him." I take a breath and follow behind. Doc introduces us and asks the women if it was fine if I stay and observe in the room. Both smile and nod in agreement. I am leaning against the sink near the door and the daughter, who looks my age more or less, stays standing at the left side of the bed that her father is lying in underneath a thin off-white sheet. Her right hand is holding her dad's hand and her left is stroking his head. The mother, who looks about the same age as my mom, has taken a seat next to Doc on the right side of the bed. "How are you doing?" Doc asks the mother and daughter. "Dad, you still with us?" The daughter asks loudly, "Dad, you with us?" She says it again as her father rolls to the right with his eyes closed, smiling slightly. "Thank god, you scared me!" she says. Doc leans in towards the mother and says, "I know this question is difficult, but if your husband's heart were to stop, what would you like us to do?" The mother bursts into tears. The daughter breaks away from her father's hand to walk over and give her mom a hug and a kiss on the cheek and then she walks back to clutching her father's hand. "I'm so sorry" the mother repeats to Doc. "You have nothing to be sorry for," Doc tells her while rubbing her shoulder and handing her a tissue. In a shaky voice and with tears rolling down both sides of her face, the mother looks up at Doc and says, "I don't know how I am going to answer that; I mean I don't think I am ready."

"I understand. Let us give you some time alone together and we be back in to check in a little bit," Doc softly says. The mother nods yes in agreement. "Dad, you with us?" the daughter asks. "Dad! Dad! You with us? Come on Dad, please stay with us!" The daughter yells as we start walking out. I made eye contact with the mother and daughter as I made a turn towards the door, trying to say something, but my lips remained locked closed. My expression felt so weird, so cold and so wrong. Who was I right now? A daughter? A sister? A friend? A researcher? How would it change the way I was standing, the way I was breathing and the way I left the room, should I have enacted another role? I walked out as a researcher and it felt so disconnected, so shallow to do at this moment. What I wanted to do was give them both a hug and tell them how sorry I was that they were going through this. Doc sat down at the computer and I grabbed my bag. Looking at her I said, "I am taking off, thank you for letting me shadow today." "Really? Everything okay?" she asks. "Yeah,

I am ok. See you Sunday." I walk out the glass doors, not realizing what I had done until exiting the highway on my way home: I had left. More importantly, I could leave. Doc had to stay and be with patients for another two hours to complete her eight plus-hour shift. She couldn't leave or even go get some fresh air in that moment like I could. And the family in bed one, they couldn't leave either.

Caring individuals and organizations, like hospice and the emergency department, manage symptoms that aren't always visible but are arguably the most important at any stage of life. Further, these organizations were developed to respond to some of our deepest fears in life: losing control, feeling pain, and being lonely. They were designed, in some way or another, based on the belief that there is something therapeutic in intentionally listening to patients' stories and suffering, as if some degree of pain can be managed through words.

Although the belief in the therapeutic effect of listening to a patient's suffering has not changed, our way of responding to suffering and aging individuals has.

This book is about caring for each other throughout life, and especially around the end of life. It shares with others a sensitive account of the difficult and, at times, tragic moments around aging and illness. And it wants to go further, to account for the day-to-day ways of talking and the way sense is made within these settings. I want to be able to capture the voices of providers, patients, and families in their own moments of trying to understand and talk to each other, and me, about real events that occur in their lives.

The book is a journey. It starts with the out-of-control feelings I had when I first entered the emergency department and hospice and started being a part of these day-to-day experiences, not having a vocabulary to understand them. From there, I will share what the literature says about making sense of end of life, and what some of our best theories tell us about understanding what otherwise would be incomprehensible moments. We will hear from providers themselves about what it is like working in these settings, what they say and what they do in order to bring control to difficult situations. In doing so, we will see how these two distinct sites organize care in a way that provides incredible opportunities for communicating around end of life, and also the tremendous complexity around our ability to make decisions that match the feelings and wishes of those we love, and those who love us.

· 1 ·

DYING IN THE 21ˢᵀ CENTURY

Almost a third of the money spent by Medicare—about $66.8 billion a year—goes to chronically ill patients in the last two years of life. Medicare, the federal health insurance program insuring 47 million elderly and disabled Americans, helps to pay for hospital and physician visits, prescription drugs, and other acute and post-acute services (Centers for Medicare and Medicaid Services, 2010; Department of Health and Human Services Center for Medicare & Medicaid Services, 2013).

More than 90 million Americans live with at least one chronic illness, and seven out of ten Americans die from chronic disease (Dartmouth Atlas, 2010). As chronic disease progresses, the amount of care delivered and the costs associated with this care increase dramatically. Patients with chronic illness in their last two years of life, for example, account for about 32% of total Medicare spending, with much of it going toward physician and hospital fees associated with repeated hospitalizations (Medicare Part A and Part B). Further, 16% of the gross national product (GNP) is spent on healthcare, and this number is expected to rise to 20% by 2015 (Centers for Medicare and Medicaid Services, 2010; Department of Health and Human Services Centers for Medicare & Medicaid Services, 2013). This statistic is two times higher than other nations, and the U.S. ranks 40ᵗʰ in quality indicators.

In 2000, 35 million American people were 65 and older. Between longer life spans and aging baby boomers, the population of Americans aged 65 years or older will double during the next 25 years to roughly 72 million. And by 2030, older adults will account for roughly 20% of the population (CDC, State of Aging & Health in America, 2012). Advances in medical technology and disease prevention in combination with the aging of the population have resulted in dramatic growth in the number of adults living with serious illness (Morrison et al., 2008). And despite a considerabe amount of effort and expenditures, patients with serious illness receive poor quality medical care: unmet personal care needs, untreated symptoms, caregiver burden, low family and patient satisfaction, and enormous costs (Morrison et al., 2008).

In fiscal year 2007, $2.2 trillion dollars were spent on healthcare, and Medicare spending is expected to increase from $426 in 2007 to $844 billion in 2017 (Department of Health and Human Services Centers for Medicare & Medicaid Services, 2013). Even more, the Congressional Budget Office predicts that the cost of long-term care will reach $207 billion in 2020 and $346 billion in 2040 (Congressional Budget Office, 1999; Department of Health and Human Services Centers for Medicare & Medicaid Services, 2013).

Contradictions with end-of-life care have been widely recognized for years. Specifically, the use of palliative medicine and hospice care has increased. So too have discussions of prognosis and goals of care, leading to reduced spending, reduced utilization of unnecessary tests, and improved quality of life (Goodman, Villareal, & Jones, 2010). Although healthcare still falls short of the care that most patients want to receive, and providers want to give, health care for elderly Americans at the end of life is changing. However, our language for talking about treatment options and patient preferences around the end of life is taking longer to change and develop.

This book carefully details the way language shapes decisions around end-of-life care. The emergency department and hospice provide emergency care and end-of-life care, respectively, in Colorado. The patients, families, and providers come from diverse populations with diverse forms of knowledge. Together, they exemplify the formal and informal contexts, language, and strategies for organizing care around life and death. These sites have similarities and profound differences. Their juxtaposition illustrates common themes around language use and presents microcosms of the larger health care system. Both sites have drastically different cultures, climates, rhythms, and purposes for providing care. The themes from both will serve as guidance and reflection for other areas of caregiving.

Essentially, the way we talk about life and death has consequences and opportunities for the way we feel, think, and act with respect to care and aging. I am working to answer questions surrounding the production of meaning as it is a way of representing and presenting a culture by describing and understanding localized practices, particularly communicative practices. Ethnography is well equipped to aid this examination. Understanding these practices helps me to uncover how talk produces and reproduces certain meanings, norms, and strategies around the end of life.

Life is fragile and, more often than not, life is not fair. People die—young, old and not-so-old—every minute of every day. We die cold and we die warm. We also die immediately, unexpectedly, and perhaps over an extended period of time. We die with family and friends around and we also die alone, something I am afraid of. Often, we are not sure how we want to die nor have much idea how others wish to die. And sometimes, we talk more about a person's life when we realize they're dying than we do when they are living.

Even more, we tread deeply in language that both constrains and enables our understanding of life and death.

Words do things for us: they make us feel, they make us think, they help us reason, they take us places, they hurt us, and they also heal us. For these reasons, there is tremendous struggle around meaning, interpretation, and communication at the end of life. We struggle to make sense of the dying process. We struggle to understand how we should live in order to have a peaceful death. We struggle with what people say and what people hear around the dying process. We struggle interpreting the significant costs and spending associated with the end of life. We struggle interpreting what a hospital and hospice are like, and what they should be like. We struggle interpreting the significance of our lives as well as the lives of others. We struggle making decisions about how to live, and of course, how to die. We struggle making decisions about what kind of care we should receive, or what kind of care we can afford or have access to.

We also struggle communicating with people who are dying. What words do we have available to us? What words help in these situations? What words hurt us in these situations? Are my doctors talking to each other to coordinate my care? Are my patients listening to my care plan? Will my insurance cover this treatment? And we struggle with saying too much or not being able to say enough to someone who is dying. Therefore, end of life is a subject that is significant to all of us because the decisions we make—and the decisions made for us—have significant social, economic, political, physical, and emotional costs.

In order to understand how communication is critical to understanding end of life, I will introduce the sites throughout the pages so that you may begin to get a feeling, as I did, for what they are like. You will hear from the providers themselves through narratives and actual interviews. But it is important to note that what you hear will be a representation of what they actually said, since you in fact were not there and therefore, it is unfair for me to believe that you will hear them in the same way I have. In addition to hearing providers, you will also hear my own voice describe what it felt like being there. Beginning to feel what it is like in these places will give you an understanding of the complexity of these spaces, the vocabularies used in these places, the events that take place. Moreover, it will give you a feeling for what it is like to work in these places, and a feeling for what it is like to be a patient in these places.

Because after all, the way we feel is inherently connected to the language we use and to the many ways language uses us. That said, you will hear two voices throughout this project: one voice trying to understand what is going on and another illustrating the consequences of talk in both of these places.

Just as important, in these sites, I was an incoherent person constantly being true to what I was hearing and also being true to the craziness I was feeling about life and death. But it is in the emotional and incoherent moments where I understood the most and gained tremendous insight. My feelings of craziness and incoherence in these sites give a detailed sense of what often gets hidden behind protocols, algorithms, and routines in order to control the uncomfortable rhythms that beat within their domains.

Behind the glass doors and windows of both sites, hidden mostly from public view, are the workers, providers, families, and patients who bear witness to the pain and suffering of death as well as the joy and hope of life. And behind these glass doors, I have met intelligent, compassionate, and humble people. Providers, who endlessly inflict pain in the name of healing, are the bearers of hope, and the messengers of death serve extremely emotional roles when embraced at these places (Hirschmann, 1999). And providers who work every day in the face of life and death speak through voices, interactions, norms, stories, realities, and experiences that are rarely questioned and deeply misunderstood by many of us on the outside. Together, they provide an important picture of what it means to live and die in the 21st century and the challenges and opportunities of coordinating care around the end of life.

My purpose is to understand these stories about life and death to give readers a chance to learn as I did, listening to patients, providers, and family members speak for themselves. Additionally, I focus on language use to understand the ways in which language produces care experiences around the end of life. Even more, I focus on how individuals use language to expose how implicit values are shaping choices and decisions around end of life. Values are not simply beliefs or attitudes that someone holds and possesses. Rather, "to value is to differentiate—to act, choose, or desire. To differentiate is to stratify, not by holding one differentiated thing over the other but by differentiating along this line rather than another" (Deetz, 1992, p. 61).

This book provides no solutions, answers, or panacea to dying or living with illness. Rather, my goal is twofold. First, I will use insights from different positions to build an intuitive way of talking about communication that enables the reader to rethink the processes of interacting with others around the end of life. Second, I will attend to the subtle processes of meaning and decision production to disrupt common ways of talking and interacting around end of life, thereby bringing contestation to a set of practices that are both constraining and enabling patients', providers', and families' ability to talk differently, and have some choice in the meanings surrounding life and death. Because this project is proposed more as a window on clinical life than an overview of the medical field, it is written in a way that should be accessible to academics, providers, patients, and families.

The Changing Landscape Concerning End of Life

Rapid changes in the organization of U.S. medical care and technology have altered the communicative contexts in which patients, families, and providers make their decisions and coordinate care around end of life. Discourses of death and dying have consequences for how individuals interact and make decisions in everyday life (Seale, 1998). Discourses also provide and organize a variety of narratives and discursive resources for dying and bereaved people to interpret their situations, as well as for those providing care.

This book examines how clinical settings such as an emergency department and a hospice both encourage and stifle discourses about what it means to live and die, and the ways in which these discourses intersect with the unique circumstances of an individual's life and health. Moreover, this book focuses on how we as a society engage in language and discourses designed to transform an orientation towards death into one that embraces life. My hope is to understand how delicately balanced discourses are organized in managing life both in terms of quantity and quality of days.

The language of an emergency department and a hospice often is considered to involve two voices—emergency and hospice medicine. Even so, the claim that there are only *two* discourses, like "clinical" and "curative," is highly problematic because embedded in care settings is a conglomeration of discourses about relieving pain and the inherent disparity of saving and ending a life. This opposition, however, is largely accepted and rarely interrogated. Even more rarely interrogated is the very complexity of language and human interaction. Therefore, in this study I move from our everyday normative and rational impressions of how to talk, or how others should talk around end of life, to an in-depth look at the complexity of talk and the unique ways language is used around end of life.

In what follows, two medical providers share their accounts of working in end-of-life care in contemporary times. This is another move—or invitation—for you to step in and begin to get a feel for these places. The narratives are cleaned up to be read as stories, but the words belong to the providers. The words in bold are my verbatim interview questions. After each narrative, I include my own voice or reflection describing the sites when I first arrived in order to share my own attitudes and assumptions from the outset and how they evolved over time.

Gerry is a nurse practitioner at a hospice. She has reddish shoulder-length hair parted on the side and rectangle-shaped wire glasses. She has soft wrinkles around her eyes and a very warm, soothing voice. She smiles a lot and wears a huge green hospice lanyard around her neck with a fistful of keys. She was holding her flip cell phone and a stack of papers when we met. We sat at a small laminate coffee table in the hospice kitchen. Three other tables were occupied by patients, visitors, and staff and hummed with white noise. The ice machine was grinding in front of me and metal trays of plates and silverware were stacked on a dolly while a woman removed each tray and hosed off the plates, placing them on another metal tray to dry. Behind Gerry was a five-foot-wide fish tank with artificial coral and several colorful fish swimming in circles as the filter bubbled and gurgled. Gerry was drinking a hot Chai tea in a white mug she had taken from the coffee machine in the kitchen and the smell of black Folgers coffee you inhale at any diner was all I could smell. I had a glass of water in a clear plastic cup with no ice. In the following narrative, she describes the challenges and gratifications of her work in general and the language of hospice in particular.

What's a bad day here? *Well a bad day is when I can't help somebody in the sense that they don't seem to understand what I am saying or maybe the team isn't able to communicate effectively—I mean that is really one of the key challenges with our role is what we say and what people hear. And if we are speaking different languages, which can often happen at the end of life, then poor communication is going to make for a really bad day. And it happens in all different shapes and sizes. Each situation is going to be different but if you have a day where you are just not able to communicate openly with another person, it's going to make for a really bad day.*

What do you mean by different languages? *Could be a cultural difference. Could be just a knowledge deficit about their disease process. It could be in the form of—maybe they are just in a different place of their illness, their journey—they might have an expectation that is not aligned with hospice necessarily. Not everyone comes to hospice knowing what hospice is or understanding what hospice does, or being ready for hospice. So we're not here, I'm not here to make them ready but to meet them where they're at and to see how I can help them best. And that may be staying here on hospice or it may be finding what's in line with their particular goals and values.*

What's important for this kind of work? *First and foremost, you are a human being so don't forget you are a human being! You have to be genuine. I would say listen to other people as much as you can and when you find that you are not able to interact with people anymore whether it is on that given day or that you have* to take care of yourself or you're never going to be able to take care of other people. So care for yourself, be genuine.

You have to be really empathetic. You have to be very compassionate. You absolutely have to have a good heart, which probably encompasses all of the above. I would say the primary characteristic that you really need is to be an empathetic person. But at the same time you have to realize that this is the patient's and family's experience and not your experience. So that they—the patient and the family—are essentially the ones that are going through this and you are trying to guide them.

Are there any barriers that get in the way trying to guide patients and families? Yes, in fact, the day-to-day nonsense I like to call it, just the interruptions, the flow of events, and the work environment. Essentially, when I talk or meet with a patient and the family, I try to immerse myself in that experience and really close everything else out and not be thinking about what else I could be doing whether it's with another patient or whether it is something personal, to really give 100% when I am with that patient.

Because being a nurse to me is something really special. It is something that is very personal, it's just a very unique relationship that you have with another individual that you aren't always able to share in other locations or professions. And it's something that, being a nurse, to me it's more about, it's not just the medical piece or the health piece—it's really relating to that person in a way where they feel open enough to disclose things that are very personal and private issues. And you have to earn their trust, you have to earn their relationship, you have to, you know, just because I am a nurse doesn't mean you have to tell me everything about you.

Are there specific things that you do with patients? Yes, of course. I try to just get to know the person. It's hard because there is a blur between personal and professional, but I try and engage the individual just talking with them, not just coming in and focusing on the issue at hand. I mean if I come in and say how is your breathing today? If that is going to be the extent of my relationship with a person, then that is probably how they are going to disclose things to me, reveal things to me and that's all our relationship is going to be. For hospice, where we all wear multiple hats and even though I assume the medical provider/nursing piece of their care, I can't shut them down if they want to talk about something else because that is not what it is all about. So I essentially just try and get to know that person, try to get to know what they are comfortable revealing to me and go from there.

Hospice care is difficult and people often don't have a good sense of what it is. **How come?** Well, there is a real interest coupled with fear. It's a real conversation stopper at times. There are a lot of people that just say, "oooohhhh." My family and friends will still ask me, but there is still kind of a veil that comes over them when *they talk with me about how are things at hospice, their voice changes and it's serious stuff and I realize in conversation with them how open I have become to talking about dying and the end of life and how comfortable I am on a professional level with discussing dying and end of life issues.*

Do they understand what you really do? *A lot of times, for example, my family and friends will ask me exactly what I do and they have an accurate impression. My brother, he doesn't live in town and he has known that I have worked as a nurse practitioner at hospice and he kind of skirts the issue a little bit. You know I don't think he fully understands what I do.*

Why do you think this problem exists? *I think a lot of it is very emotionally charged. You know each and every one of us has known someone who has died and for most people it kind of elicits a painful emotion, probably a mixture of feelings. And so when people talk about dying, especially if they don't have the professional perspective, it becomes a very personal event and it's kind of, they may be respectful, they may feel a lot of gratitude towards hospice professionals either in the past but for a lot of people it really isn't a pleasant experience so it is something that makes them very emotional and not necessarily in a good way.*

My reflective experience: The smells of bedsores and Clorox burn my eyes and penetrate the back of my throat as I enter hospice. The hall is wide, big enough for two wheelchairs. Walking along the gray carpet by each room below the artificial flower arrangement over the patient's name and room number, I look in each room hesitantly before turning my head quickly when making eye contact with patients and family members. Why did I catch many of their eyes so frequently? Why did I feel so much resistance looking at these patients, these people, and these individuals? How could I walk by without looking at them? Was I contributing to their own objective and stigmatized position of being a hospice patient?

Attempting to understand end of life communication, why was it so hard to look, feel, hear, and smell what interests me so much? Maybe the only thing these patients want is for someone not to think something is wrong with them, that they can't be looked at, touched, or talked to? Maybe talking and listening to them was exactly what we both needed? What if that was me or my family and someone walked by or jerked their head suddenly when they caught my eye during a time of great uncertainty in one's life? Transitioning through a system that deals with patients and their identities by bed numbers, scores, and results, how was I enacting a new form of identity? What would it be like to die if people were essentially trained to value dying instead of being unimpressed by the fragility of life itself.

Now, begin to step in and get a feeling for the emergency department as Susan, an emergency physician, shares her experiences. We met at her house in Denver and sat in the living room that looks out on a quaint city street with dog walkers and joggers. She has short brown hair, freckles, and large hazel eyes with flashes of green tint. She has bright white teeth that light up her face when she smiles. She was wearing blue scrubs and a gray half-zip sweater when we met because she had just arrived from a Physical Therapy appointment after her shift at the emergency department. When she sat down on the sofa, one of her Labradors jumped on her lap and the other found a spot on her foot. She was eating a Stonyfield fruit yogurt shortly into the interview, feeding herself, and then offering a lick off the spoon to both dogs. Here she describes the challenges and gratifications of her work in general and the language of emergency medicine in particular.

It's like a job like everyone else's job. You know you pack your lunch, hoping you get a few minutes to eat in peace. I mean, it's just weird, you know sometimes a patient will die and a minute later we are ordering pizza and it's not that we have disregard for that person's life, it's that—that's our job and it's no different from the guy who is a car mechanic where it is tragic for the car owner whose transmission fell out, who can't afford to replace it and that car is dead. Yeah, you say, but we're talking about a life. I get that but everything is still a job and you don't want us—I mean what are you going to do, someone dies in the ER and everyone has to go home because they are so emotionally distraught so we have to bring in a whole new crew? That is a hard thing for people to get. It's not that we are not compassionate—we've been doing it for 20 years and our job goes on. As soon as you finish with this one person who died and console their family, now you are 15 people behind and they are all mad as hell at you.

What makes for a good day at work? *I think the personalities in the ER— different nurses, and other docs you are working with—is definitely one of the bigger variables. If you've got the right mix, everyone has good energy, it's funny, sarcastic, playful, and we can diffuse a patient's energy with each other. The patients that wear us down are the patients that are demanding, have ridiculous expectations, like I have had this for 15 years and I have seen 10 specialists and I am here Friday night at 10 pm and I expect you to have an answer to why this is going on. That can be absurd and sometimes you can let it roll off you but sometimes patients are so in your face and make you in your weak moments really defensive and engage that behavior and that makes for a bad shift.*

And then there are other things in the mix that make for a bad shift—last night it was a bad shift because there were a lot of patients that had a lot of sad diagnoses, like one woman came in, had breast cancer 15 years ago, she had bilateral mastectomies, they didn't recommend chemo and radiation, they said it was not called for it was such a small tumor. And she comes in with a complaint of a herniated disc kind of symptoms and has enough neurological symptoms that I did an MRI because she had lost her reflex, she had lost some bladder control, and sometimes that means you have to do something surgical. Got an MRI and she had boney metastases throughout...and you know it was like taking all the wind out of her sail and I think she thought it was never something she'd ever worry about that came back...you know that is hard, it's hard to give somebody that diagnosis, it's hard to feel like in the ER you're doing anything but dumping all this horrible information on them saying, alright, why don't you follow up with your doctor, we need the bed, there's 15 more in the waiting room.

You know it's like you can't spend enough time with them—you know it's not like they need you to spend more time with them that minute because they need some time to take it all in and sort it out, but the ER seems like a funny place to be handing out that info. So, bad diagnoses can wear us down because we are people too you know and we have our own fears about getting illnesses or it might remind you of a friend you had that had something and it just sometimes gets really personal and it's hard to keep up your defenses and it's not to say that you are like a wall and impervious to all that is around you but I don't know that people get that. At some level we have to have the wall up or we would be consumed by horrific diagnoses and sadness and other stuff we do.

Having to try and save someone's life while family are wailing right next to you, is not an easy task. You have to somewhere put it aside and though you know it hurts—you're trying to help somebody and I guess that is the hardest part that in medicine, at some point you have to figure out how to manage it and if you don't find a way to let it out later it starts to make you a bitter, cynical, burned out doctor that takes it out on people and that is the end result that patients see and say what an ass that doc is, but they might not appreciate all the pain and suffering we've had to bear witness to that has taken its toll on us, even though we signed up for it. It still is hard and they don't teach us how to manage that. And there are conferences and lectures on how to handle the difficult patient or whatever but it is not really something we embrace. You know it's not like, hey look what I am going to. It's more you take it on because somewhere down the line you learn you've got to do these things to save yourself.

My reflective experience: Red phone rings as Kelly, a nurse, walks out of the break room. It rings a second time as she picks up the phone in her left hand while simultaneously opening the pen with her right hand that is attached to the dry erase board above the phone. "ER," she states. And begins writing the symbol for female, 58, and then two other codes I didn't recognize. "Ok, we'll have a bed ready for her when she arrives," she says and hangs up the phone.

Doc, eating edamame and Rice Krispie treats, swivels around, glances at the board and then around to me and says, "that'll be a good one for you."

Oh no, I think. How could she know that much from those two simple codes on the white board? "Why?" I ask.

"She drowned and has no pulse," she says.

I sigh again as three nurses make their way into bed two, removing and changing lines, preparing IVs, and activating monitors. Brent's voice, a triage nurse, comes over the intercom saying, "ambulance arrival bed two, ambulance arrival bed two." I am standing near Doc's computer as the stretcher comes around the corner. Bypassing the two EMTs pushing the stretcher, my eyes look at the patient, whose face is Smurf purple, ringed with wet hair, but I could still make out gray tints of color. Her eyes were closed and her mouth was slightly open, with several blankets over her, even as her purple right foot popped out from under the blanket. Several nurses are already in bed two waiting as two more walk in following the stretcher, then another doc and the pediatrician on call at the time follow behind. And with a push from Doc on my upper back, I trickle in last and stand near the back of the room.

The EMTs start giving their report as the blankets are pulled off of her body and one nurse starts attaching one of those sticky monitors to her left breast, her right breast, and two on her abdomen. At this point, the woman is completely naked and purple. The nurses continue to move their hands on, in, and around her. The monitor lights up with a zero in the top right and the light, which is usually going up and down, is simply moving horizontally across. A different nurse places the tube in the urethra, just above the vaginal opening. She continues to push the woman's layers of skin away from the area so that she can clean and insert the tube. The woman is still completely exposed. Was she dead? What happened to her? A third nurse has connected oxygen with a mask over it so the woman now has a tube from her bladder, a tube in her nose, one in her mouth, and four monitors on her upper and lower chest within minutes. Lastly, warm blankets are layered over her body including a heating blanket that looks like a raft.

"What's her temp?" one of the docs asks from behind.

"14," a nurse replies. (This is Celsius, equivalent to about 55 degrees).

"Do we have another heating blanket we can put directly on her body and leave the one on top?" the doc asks again.

A nurse walks briskly out and comes back with another heating blanket. A tech standing next to me looks over at me and asks, "Are you doing alright?"

"Yeah, thanks. Is she dead?"

"Well," he said, "she is too cold for us to resuscitate or pronounce her dead." Completely confused, I stare at him. He says, "They say you're not dead till you're warm and dead." "What?" I respond.

"Yeah, it's complicated, but the body must be 32 degrees before we can do anything."

Not dead till you're warm and dead I kept saying to myself. Who are these people doing this work? What goes on in their minds, their hearts, and their souls when they go home at night or early in the morning? How do they do this?

These stories—and my reflections and reactions—are filled with the tensions, the expectations, the devastations, and the compassion of coordinating care. Even more, the stories represent the changing communicative contexts in which patients, families, and providers reweave the meaning of life and death and reorganize how decisions are made around end of life. It is impossible for you to feel exactly the things I felt, but the important thing is to hold on to what it's like to work here, and to experience these places.

Attitudes Toward Death and Dying

The factors that contribute to our culture's handling of serious illness, suffering, and death can be overwhelming. Many believe that our society is "death denying." This idea has become widespread, reflected and produced in mass media where death itself has become taboo, or the "elephant in the room" (Seale, 1998). It is also supported by the well-known story "*The Death of Ivan Ilyich*" (Tolstoy, 1886), which underscored how the medicalization of death makes death an alien experience, as no one—neither his family members nor his physician—acknowledged he was dying. Instead, those around him continued to believe that he was only sick. Ivan's daily activity becomes routine and discouraging and he believes he is surrounded by artificiality. As a result, he dies alone in his agony but experiences extreme joy as he stretches out and dies. Additionally, Callahan (2000), a leading critic of the American way of death, describes the tension between fighting death and accepting death because the United States, more than many cultures, is a death-avoidant culture or a culture committed to survival and saving lives at all costs (Cassell, 2004). Most people know that most health care dollars are spent at the first and last 30 days of life, underscoring the real cost of our fears and the natural tendency of budget fixers to look at these costs. The emotional tolls of these lengthy deaths do not go unnoticed.

Discourses of death as taboo and death as alien give rise to the construction of the reality of death. And these constructions give rise to meanings of death but also to the everyday practices through which death is handled. Charmaz (1980) argues that these perspectives are embedded with values that shape and are shaped by our own experience as well as others' experience with death and dying. The values we hold about death and dying are changing the way many of us experience death. Even more, advances in medicine and medical technology have changed the way in which Americans are dying.

Quick and intense deaths caused by infectious disease, accident, or injury are no longer common (Callahan, 2000) with sudden death being responsible for 10% of deaths and chronic illness being responsible for 90% of deaths (CDC, 2009). As Ragan, Wittenberg-Lyles, Goldsmith, & Sanchez-Reilly (2008, p. 5) state, "The preeminence of medical science and advanced technology, which have led to the eradication of many diseases once considered death sentences, permit us the belief that we have conquered death, that it is no longer the inevitable, natural conclusion to life."

Callahan (2000) summarizes that medical science and advanced technology have resulted in longer lives and worse health, longer illnesses and slower deaths, and longer aging and increased dementia. In essence, the medical process of dying has replaced the act of death. As a result of the changing contexts in which we die, Americans are experiencing death differently today than in the previous century. Of the 2.3 million deaths that occurred in 1995, more than two-thirds were older than 70. Additionally, as more causes of death result from chronic conditions, people are living in a dying role longer, thereby increasing the necessity for communicating more frequently with dying persons (Bern-Klug & Chapin, 1999). This necessity ultimately generates difficult problems in the way we live our lives and the way we make decisions around how we want to live and die (Callahan, 2000).

How and when do you want to die? How much pain and suffering will you be willing to bear, and at what cost? What do you owe others when you die? These questions grow out of a larger fear of death and highlight how talking about death affects the way people communicate with and about a person who has a terminal illness. In fact, the presence of someone who is dying can be uncomfortable on both an individual and social level, creating great apprehension with the dying during a process that is undoubtedly intimate for families of a dying person and for providers caring for the dying (Littlewood, 1993). Apprehension is also produced through the ways individuals talk about death and dying. According to Corr (1997) as cited in Ragan, Wittenberg-Lyles, Goldsmith & Sanchez-Reilly (2008, p. 7):

> Prominent illustrations of ways in which death is forbidden in much of modern society include language of ordinary discourse, professional speech and communication about dying. It is important to pay attention to these linguistic practices because naming helps to define and to determine reality. How we speak says a good deal about who we are and the attitudes we hold…(p. 36).

The phrases, for example, "not dead till they are warm and dead," "next stop, heaven,"…"letting go," "she lost her battle with cancer," "he fought until the end," "she has passed away," "he has gone to a better place," "expired," "coded," and "not till the doctor pronounces them dead" are examples of how our thoughts, reflections, and values about death and the dying process are created, maintained, and experienced.

The words, fears, struggles, and experiences shape our meanings and understandings about death. Interestingly, the shaping of these meanings is taking on new forms, thereby forcing new questions about them. Recent awareness that death causes human dilemmas has been transformed into a vision of death as the new social problem of our time. But to define death as a problem suggests that there are solutions to it. For example, many Americans today see technology as an escape from the inevitability of death and believe that technological advances will be able to fix any bodily damage created throughout their lives (Ufema, 2006).

Furthermore, in such times of uncertainty, previous recipes for handling the dilemmas that death poses are called into question, thereby encouraging us all to re-think our understandings of nature and death and ultimately of what it means to live a human life (Babrow & Mattson, 2003; Charmaz, 1980). This matters because discourses around end-of-life care have enormous emotional, physical, social, material, spiritual, and financial costs for all involved.

When I ethnographically shadowed three times per week at the ED and volunteered at hospice every week for two years, the costs amplified around two tensions. First, the tension of having everything I ever read and heard about death come in direct opposition to the reality of it. Second, the tension of trying to handle the wildness and newness of death using outdated language and processes not designed to make sense of our current situation.

· 2 ·

THE COST OF UNDERSTANDING

At the beginning, I thought the ED would be more difficult for me to experience as a researcher, a student, and a 27-year-old daughter, granddaughter, and sister. I was disgusted at times with what I saw and what I heard. But I have also been astonished with the care, courage, intelligence, compassion, and strength of patients, families, and providers in the ED. Hospice was going to be a saving grace in the messiness of death. Or so I thought. It was going to be a place of comfort, people enjoying their last moments living without needles, cords, and machines. For some reason, the loud noises and bright lights were comforting in the ED. At hospice, the silence rattled my soul up and down. I couldn't escape patients' bodies, swollen, bandaged, wrinkled, white, green, bald, blind, deaf, cold, smelly, motionless, and crippled. At hospice, I saw how illness and age literally take over bodies, skin, and minds every week.

By year one of my immersion with these sites I was breaking down. My experience of breaking down tells us much about living and language. The past few months have been spent getting even closer with my data while still remaining in the field on Friday afternoons. I've primarily been reading through fieldnotes and re-reading interview transcriptions. Writing notes from the ED came naturally: I saw, listened, and reported. But I am not sure if I ever really let myself feel what was happening when I was there. At the beginning, the smell of the ED made me want to vomit. And the artificial fluorescent lights burned into my head without me even knowing it. I put lavender under my nose and on my wrists every time I entered the ED for the first few months and drove with the windows down, despite the weather, across Hospital Blvd. to Ellsworth until I was on the highway.

The disinfectant that scoured the floors tingled my nose. The excessive Purell squirted on every one's hands, foaming in and out after each patient, became a saving grace as I found myself doing the same: squirting sanitizer into my palms, rubbing my palms together bringing my hands to my nose, and taking a deep inhale. Consequently, smelling rubbing alcohol became a useful trick to minimize the other and more indelicate odors. Perhaps the smell of alcohol so close to my nose, temporarily, impaired my ability to smell. Interestingly, I became immune to this smell and the irritable sound of beeps and bells that orchestrate every second in the ED. Even more, I grew impervious to most patients and most conversations when I was there. In a sense, I had developed my own form of armor for being present. Yes, I ran out on occasion or burst in to tears when I left the ED and was alone in my car. I thought every hour I was there how fortunate it was that I, or someone I knew, was not in bed one, bed two, bed three, or bed four.

Reading my notes a year later, I am taken aback that I was there and saw the things and heard the things I reported. And so too, that everyone around me saw and heard the same things but through different eyes. In the ED, patient ailments range from a stubbed toe to a fractured foot, cuts, bruises, chronic headaches, liver disease, kidney disease, HIV, and terminal cancer. But patients never stayed long when I was there. Patients were either admitted into the hospital, went home, or died. In any case, the ED rarely saw them again, except for those they referred to as "frequent flyers" (Gawande, 2009).

The patients I saw die, died quickly. For example, one patient came in with hardly any pulse and freezing. He couldn't say anything and therefore his Power-Of-Attorney (POA) spoke for him. The resident on duty knew that time was precious and continued to ask what his wishes were if his heart were to stop. The resident said, "should we do everything possible? Or should we let him die without trying to save him?" "Let's try once more," his POA said. And that is what the doctors and nurses did when his heart stopped. The patient died the next morning.

Another time I arrived to the ED and stood in my usual spot, and the unruly mess of bed one literally created its own mess in my stomach. Monitors were on the ground, sheets that looked like they had been ripped off were lying half on the bed and half on the floor, wrappers from IVs were covering the tile around the bed, and cords were draped over and under the bed.

"What happened in bed one?" I asked. "Patient coded and didn't survive," the tech said quietly to me. For many in the ED, a messy room is symbolic of a "fair death," meaning the team did everything they could. In other words, the messier the room, the harder they worked to save a life. These situations in the ED happened too often and too quickly for me to understand in the moment. But one thing was clear: I was ready to see how death was understood and dealt with in another place. In between transitioning sites, I contacted Dr. Jones, a palliative care physician, to get her opinion on where I needed to be to get a better understanding of death and life in medical settings. She invited me to observe a daylong palliative care round while she organized a visit to hospice, which was her recommendation for where I should go next. I observed palliative care rounds at Denver Peak Hospital and was mystified by the harmony that occurred when a team consisting of one doctor and two nurses went from bed to bed, spending a minimum of 45 minutes with each patient. The care seemed genuine and a way to bring comfort and tranquility to a patient who was dying. They knew so much about every patient. For example, they knew that when Laura was crocheting, it meant she was feeling better. Laura, tan skin with short wavy dark hair, didn't have her needle and yarn out the day I visited, which meant she was in a lot of pain. She cried when the team was there and begged them not to leave if she fell asleep. Her belly was swollen and her face puffy as her eyes dragged between opening and closing. Dr. Jones held her right hand, staring into her eyes. Helen, one of the other nurses, held her left hand, also gazing into her eyes. Joan, the other nurse, had her hands placed on Laura's ankles, gently massaging them.

This level of care astonished me. Feeling refreshed after seeing it, I felt ready to see what goes on at hospice and why several doctors and nurses thought I needed to spend time there if I was ever going to understand death and dying. Dr. Jones gave me directions to hospice but I had some trouble finding it. As I got near, I called the receptionist three times.

"Turn on Ellis Lane," she kept saying.

Below Ellis Lane is a sign, "No Outlet." Two tired-looking apartment complexes with covered windows, people smoking on the stoops, and balconies with signs advertising reduced rent, lined both sides of the street before the hospice, which was at the end of the street. The chapel was first, on the left, and then two cream-colored buildings with several low windows. The

American flag waved gently above the parking lot and bird feeders lined each room's window, some stocked with seeds and some not. There was a smoking lounge at the east entrance and gas-lit fireplaces in both lobbies of the single-story buildings.

I met Gerry, the nurse practitioner, at hospice Wednesday morning at 8 am. Dr. Jones had suggested I spend three full days to get a feel for things. Gerry and I talked about my motivations for coming, as well as her role at the hospice, at a table in the kitchen. We sat in the west side kitchen at a wooden table with a plastic cloth and a carnation as the centerpiece. I immediately felt connected to Gerry. She invited me to put my bag and lunch in her office before we started the day checking in with patients. Gerry moved slowly between each room, and so did everyone at hospice.

The lights were much dimmer at hospice than in the ED but the smell that I later became impervious to was back. The carpet was a dark gray and the halls entrapped me. The scary stillness of death was new for me. The ED felt like a happy playground compared to here. Gerry's office was in the nurses' station, in a dark and small corner office. Articles about caregiving and burnout hung from the doors and cubicle dividers. The nurses' station was closed off by big glass windows—the standard kind of window often at doctors' offices that slide open when someone approaches and slide closed when they leave. We had lunch together that day and the following day with Dr. Jones, the medical director at hospice, who rode her bike to work. They asked me how things were going but I didn't have much to share except that the hospice was new to me and I never imagined it would be so different from the ED.

Two days went by with Gerry, but I couldn't return for day three. I felt terribly sick and remember driving home wondering if I should pull over or whether I could make it home. I emailed Gerry that night, telling her that I wouldn't be there in the morning because I wasn't feeling well. She wrote me an email and called telling me how much she appreciated me not pushing myself to return and that every one of us handles being there differently, so it's important to listen to your body. I did listen to my body and didn't go back for a month. Then I decided to interview Gerry to talk about her experiences, training, and so on. We met at 8 am and sat in the kitchen again, on the east side, next to the fish tank with the loud filter. A family of three sat a few tables away for an admissions interview and the kitchen staff was busy preparing the next meal. Gerry and I talked for over 50 minutes and it helped me to hear about her experience, and the purpose of hospice within the larger healthcare system, from her perspective. She encouraged me to volunteer there, as long I felt okay. She emphasized several times how hospice is such a special place.

After our coffee, I talked with the volunteer coordinator, who scheduled an interview the following week. My new-hire orientation was three weeks long. The training lasted two days from 8 to 5pm, lunch included. We covered several topics and heard directors describe the history of the Hospice of Saints; hospice and palliative care philosophies and concepts; complementary therapies; infection control; safety; pastoral services; social services; cultural care; dietary-comfort kitchen; death and dying; bereavement; communication; and pain management. Slowly, I began to share the vision of hospice held by Gerry and many who walked the halls, that hospice is a really wonderful place. A week later, I started my six hours of floor training, pushing the hospitality cart. Two weeks after that, I started my new job every Friday afternoon from 3 to 5 pm. I went in to every room except those where patients were being bathed, were sleeping, were "on watch," or had visitors. Many of the patients seemed to enjoy talking to me and wondered why someone my age would volunteer there. After each shift, in white three-ring binders, we had to document what patients had to drink, what they had to eat, and anything interesting or unusual about their mood. This took me almost an hour every time I was there.

At the end of each log is the patient's information: date of birth, religious views, primary physician, address, admitted from, family names, and diagnosis. And sometimes there was a small paragraph describing their childhood. Many of their histories were sad for me, without an address and without family members or a power of attorney (POA). Many were from foster families, many had their own young kids, and many were young themselves—20 and 29—and as old as 98. Every Friday brought new patients, meaning some had died or gone home, wherever and whatever that meant for them. By a year later, before I knocked to enter each room on Fridays, things at hospice began to wear on me. What was wearing, I'm not sure, but I was overwhelmed with the patients' unending pain and suffering.

The nurses I interviewed and the training I went through reiterated the naturalness of death and in many cases, the beauty of a "good and peaceful" death. Did these patients know that when they came to hospice, at least someone was certain they were going to die, and die pretty soon for that matter? What is it like to hear that from someone? What does it feel like to come to hospice as a patient? I continued opening ginger ale cans and bags of Doritos for patients, walking a fine line between opening the can or bag of chips and letting patients do it themselves, knowing their mobility skills were declining, yet also aware that opening a can, a straw, a bag of chips was one of the only things they could control.

I started having bizarre dreams at night. They weren't about dying or hospice or medicine, but just busy dreams full of activity. I started to see patients differently while hearing, in the back of my mind, that death is a peaceful and beautiful thing and that at hospice, they see God working. At hospice they embrace life. Really? Is this what life looks like when you're near the end?

What is beautiful about dying? What is beautiful about sitting in bed, looking at the TV or out the window, for five days, three weeks or eight months? What is beautiful about experiencing enormous loss—a loss of privacy, a loss of support, a loss of mobility, a loss of appetite, a loss of communication skills, a loss of memory, a loss of feeling the ground, the wind, the rain, the snow, and the sun?

What is beautiful about a slow death? What is beautiful about an immediate death? What is beautiful about eating salty and processed food and having to eat when someone serves you? What is beautiful about not being able to brush your teeth, comb your hair, remember your child's phone numbers, or remember how to even use the phone? What is beautiful about feeling like "a cattle at an auction" wondering where you will go next and if someone will accept you? What is so beautiful about wondering if your weight gain will continue to be supported by Medicare because essentially that meant you were getting better? What is beautiful about losing most, if not all, of your possessions? What is beautiful about not having a "home" to go to? What is beautiful about wondering if you are, in fact, dying? What is beautiful about seeing or hearing people squirt hand sanitizer on their palms before and after seeing you?

Last time I was at the hospice, a patient had contracted C-Diff, a toxic and infectious bacteria that can cause severe inflammation of the colon, often seen in patients who have been on powerful antibiotics. The bacteria spreads fast and typical hand sanitizers often don't work for controlling the bacteria. Therefore, anyone who comes in contact must use soap and water for 30 seconds and wear isolation gowns. Outside this patient's room was a cart filled with yellow gowns, yellow masks, and rubber gloves, which were required wear in order to enter the room. I was pushing the cart that day and wheeled by once or twice to peek in, wondering if I should "gown up" or not. Three visitors were in the room, wearing the masks, gowns, and gloves, surrounding the patient's bed. I wheeled by a third time, stopped the cart outside, caught their eyes and while pointing at the cart said, "care for anything?"

"No, thank you," the woman responded.

Did she know I was too scared to enter? Why didn't I go in? Well honestly, because I didn't want to catch the bacteria. Was this a selfish move on my part? Was it fair? How many others were taking the same approach I did? Dying here is already so lonely, not to mention when you have to wear protection to enter the room.

What is beautiful about dying alone? What is beautiful about dying here? What precisely is beautiful about dying anywhere? Even more, what is so rewarding about working in these places? How could this work feel good to people? How are they able to sleep at night, seeing six people die in one day at hospice or seeing a full code in the ED? Why isn't anyone experiencing the horror, the fear, and the confusion that I am?

In a sense, we can die at home, in transit, in the hospital or in hospice. At the ED, it now feels as though death was more real, more honest, and less painful. It happened quickly, from what I saw. Life and death are fleeting in the ED; it comes and goes fast. At hospice, it feels like life has already gone and there is only death. Do both sites approach death the same way they approach life? Who is deciding what a good death is and what a good life is? How can someone actually be trained to see the beauty of death and even believe that death is something natural that shouldn't be feared? How did I spend so much time in these places?

I don't want to die in either one of these places, nor do I want any of my family or friends to either. In fact, I wish no one would have to die this way: quick, messy, and heroic *or* long, slow, and lonely. What is the role of faith in creating a peaceful death? Can you die peacefully without believing in someone or something larger than the self? Can you work at hospice and the ED without believing in something larger than the self? How can workers stomach the pain, the morbidity of these places? I could not anymore.

Empathy is one of the key characteristics of both places. To me, empathetic people feel much for the Other. By capitalizing the O I draw attention to a set of situations or moments that fundamentally challenge who I am and what I hold to be true. The presence of Otherness is also the presence of difference. Further, it is an act of destruction of meaning that through my encounters with these sites, something challenged me so much that will never allow me to go back to the way I was. In short, Otherness is the very moment I began to see death in a way I was not able to before. Consequently, people suffer when the Other suffers.

How do care providers deal with their suffering? Are they able to? How exactly are they courageous enough to care for people who are ill and dying? How are they courageous enough to shift mindsets between someone dying, ordering pizza, and telling someone they have a terminal illness? Who is calling on them to go to these lengths to save and help others? Where do they find the courage and compassion to care for someone else, including their own self? What does it feel like to control someone's death? What does it feel like to be responsible for how, when, and if someone dies?

What happens to life when all of it disappears? Everything you ever felt, ever experienced, ever loved, ever saw, ever tasted, ever knew, ever read, ever heard, ever listened to, slowly escapes you? What is left? What does it mean if the things I take to be so important in life lose meaning at the end? What will it be like if I forget these things when I get older? What will it be like if no one cares about these things when I get older? What is left? What will it be like to die without anyone I know surrounding me? This scares me tremendously. But how do you manage these fears? What is the meaning of life if it ends this way, stuck in an uncomfortable bed, eating salty and processed food and looking out the window at a birdfeeder? Why is life so sacred? Why is death so profane? And why are both so fragile?

Many know that the ED operates at lightning speed and their purpose is to fix 'em, get 'em out, or save 'em if they can. And most everyone knows that hospice is for people who are dying and want symptom management through less aggressive treatments. For the ED, going to hospice means patients are stopping care. For hospice, coming there from a clinical setting translates to patients being cared for, for the first time in a while. People talk about "going on" hospice, or "coming off" hospice. What exactly are they going "on" or "off"? Is it similar to the tragic ride I went on and am now slowly coming off? How do meanings that surround life and death change instantly, where focus is spent on managing symptoms and bringing comfort to patients in their last moments of life, as opposed to doing everything possible to keep someone alive? How exactly does this work?

Since many patients are admitted from the hospital to hospice, how do patients and families process "stopping clinical care"? They have a terminal illness but aren't being treated, so to speak. There is no chemo, no radiation, no aggressive medications or treatment at hospice. But there is aromatherapy, pet therapy, music therapy, pastoral services, art services, pain medications, and volunteers who serve as their own form of medicine. If a patient doesn't have a strong belief system, how do they process their experience at hospice?

Likewise, how do workers process their care without a strong belief system? Do religion and spirituality prevent things from being said or from not ever being dealt with?

Religion and spirituality provide people with answers and in many cases can serve as a sense-making device for a rather complex situation and morbid experience. Do religion and spirituality provide a sense of armor for those at hospice against death and dying? Do people really see angels before they die, like they say they do? Do people really see a light before they die like they say they do? How do you move "bad energy" in a place with so much death? What do people in the ER believe in to help process their experiences?

An ambulance arrived at the ED with a patient who had coded during the ride over, but he was admitted to bed eight. I walked behind Doc and two nurses towards the room. The EMTs were transferring the older man from the stretcher to the bed while the family watched. The doc introduced herself and walked over to the patient, whose mouth was slightly open, took her stethoscope, placed it to the older man's chest, spread open his eyes, then looked at his daughter and said, "Yes, he has indeed passed. We'll leave you alone in the room, but please let us know if we can get you anything. The nurse will be in to discuss where you'd like us to take him." We left the room and we were on to the next patient. What kind of people can do this work, seriously? Why do these sites feel so similar, yet so different? Does the average person feel what I'm feeling when they go to these places?

It's never been clear why I chose this project. The only thing I can think of is that this project chose me for some reason. I have no expectations other than to understand what happens in these two sites, what is the role of communication in maintaining the purposes of both places: to heal and comfort. What would a good death look like? Is that even possible to imagine? What would effective end-of-life care look like? And is that even possible?

I had reached a place of complete engagement and started to understand that "going native" is painfully uncomfortable. Is this where the interesting stuff really happens? What if you can't stay once you get here? What if the human instrument is experiencing compassion fatigue? What if the human instrument, in fact, is not able to see, hear, and feel the world the way they did before they started this project? Where do you find the courage to go forward when you've hit rock bottom and feel as though there is nothing fair about living and dying the way many do? What is the meaning of a project that literally gets inside of you? What is the purpose of a project that makes you feel so empty, and so sad? What are you able to think, understand, say, and write when you reach a place of discomfort with the sites you've been called to for the past two years?

I went back to hospice to push the cart a full year after starting. A false fire alarm had congregated almost everyone but the patients in the main lobby. I proceeded to prepare the cart and check the chart for any updates. The stringent smell of Clorox and urine ate through my stomach.

I started in room 101, where the patient ordered a Coke. Room 102 had no request. Tom in 103 had no request either, but after I asked him if he wanted anything he nodded and said, "get your ass over here to hear that I don't want anything." I would have probably said the same thing if I was sitting there in that same bed and someone on foot offered me a soda or chips or "anything else." I looked across the hall into 104, leaving Tom's room and saw an older man, balding, mouth frozen yet open slightly, and a trach inserted in his throat with the machine working hard next to him. A nurse was filling water and I asked her if I should enter.

She shook her head, "No, I am pretty sure they just put him 'on watch.'"

I waited as she walked to the nurses' station, watching the patient breathe by himself in the dark room.

"Yes," she said. "He just went on watch." Alone I thought, again. "On watch" carries so much weight for me. Who is doing the watching? "Gosh, that's sad," I said softly, not thinking any one would hear. The nurse turned around and said, "Yeah, hopefully he'll make it through Easter." I looked back at her and said, "I hope he gets to go sooner, he doesn't look very good." "Yeah, I guess so," she said. "I'm praying for the instant car accident, train wreck and so on kind of way out."

I nodded my head and said, "Yeah, me too."

Room 105 had no request and Gretel had her usual glass of half wine and half water, although she thought it was all wine. She was folding napkins in the kitchen when I poured it for her, wearing one of her many knit caps that she always wore.

"Anything else, Gretel?"

"No, my dear. But you know that I love you, right?" she said.

I nodded again and said, "I love you too."

Rooms 107 and 112 were in the smoking lounge and wanted a beer—one had a Coors and the other a Bud Light. Room 108 was also "on watch." Room 109 never ordered anything because he has a horrible disease and a feeding tube. But his wife is always there and takes a few diet sodas and Fritos or

Cheetos. She is missing several teeth and always tells me how exhausted she is working mornings and evenings at her two jobs and coming here in the afternoons to be with her husband.

Rooms 113a and 113b were empty. Harri was in room 114. She doesn't have very good eyesight, as per the nurse's note and my own previous interaction with her. She stares at one place no matter where I walk, so it's important I start speaking as soon as I knock so she knows who is there. She is sitting on the edge of the bed watching *Ellen* on TV but doesn't want anything from the cart. The note on my chart said, "Harri is becoming confused about why she is at hospice and if she is 'dying.' Please help her process by actively listening and use open-ended questions." What question could I have possibly asked her? And what could I have said if she asked me if she were dying?

Across the hall in 115 the door was closed but the nurse walked out and said one of the visitors would love a Diet 7Up. I handed her one and wheeled the cart toward room 116, where a nurse was using a pen and pad of paper to communicate with the patient. I waited by the door and knocked quietly. The patient looked at me and then the nurse turned around and said, "Oh, no thank you."

I walked out and a visitor was walking in. "Do you care for anything," I said. She looked at me, shook her head no, and kept walking. Room 117 was empty, and so were beds 118a and 118b.

Before I walked to the west side, I stopped at the main office to see if there was any mail to be taken over. And there was, including a box of flowers. I was planning to drop the flowers and five pieces of mail off for room 203 before starting but the door was closed when I got there. I peeked in: three adults with pen and paper were surrounding the patient's bed. I caught one woman's eye; she stared at me and subtly nodded no. I scurried away and left the flowers with the nurses to deliver and put the mail on the cart. I started in 201, Joan's room, who almost always is sleeping with her mouth open and feet exposed in a pigeon-toe position. She has beautiful white hair and moist skin, and I have never heard her speak. Room 202 was empty. The visitors in 203 had finished their family meeting so I knocked, was welcomed, and handed Lee the mail. She was cutting her flowers and asked if she or any of them cared for something to drink.

"Want a gin and tonic, Lee?"

"Sure, I guess," she said. "But in a plastic cup," pointing to the one on her stand, "with a little gin and the rest tonic."

"Anything else?" I asked.

"I'd love a glass of Cabernet," one of the women said.

"Sure, I'll be back soon." I went back to the closet to get the gin, tonic, and plastic cup. I walked back and placed Lee's drink on the table and handed the wine to the visitor and walked out.

Charlotte was on the phone across the hall but not for long. She couldn't get the phone on the receiver so I walked in, moved the blankets that were blocking her angle, and she put the phone down.

"Hey Charlotte, how are ya?"

"Oh, so far so good," she said, as she always said.

"What's new?" I said.

"Nothing really, except I am so tired of people always wanting to clean me. The nurse was in here two hours ago to clean and she just came in to say she needed to clean me again. And I told her, I am not dirty, I'm tired and I want to sleep! It's like she has nothing else to do!"

"Did you tell her you don't want to be cleaned?"

"Yes, several times but no one listens and you can't do anything here, they are always cleaning me up."

"Maybe she just really likes you, Charlotte?"

She laughed. "Yeah, maybe I need to start being mean to these people so they leave me alone and stop taking advantage of me!"

Do you want a 7Up or ginger ale from the cart?"

"Yeah, 7Up sounds real good."

I opened it, put it over ice and told her I was leaving so she can sleep. She smiled and took a sip of the 7Up.

Room 205 was on watch. Room 206 was visiting with another volunteer so I kept walking. Jay in 207, a diabetic, was looking for pork skins, and asked me to please have someone get them at the market while he enjoyed the Pepsi and Fritos I had brought him. Room 208 was empty. I had mail for room 209, who was sleeping, so I left it on her table next to one of those picture frames that slideshows endless photos from a memory card. Rooms 210, 212, 214, and 216 were empty. And room 218 was on watch, with no one around. Room 220 was also empty.

Violet in room 222 was awake for one of the first times. I gave her the mail and offered her a ginger ale since her daughter has told us she likes them.

"Hi Violet, I have some mail."

"Some milk, great, sit down."

I stayed standing. "How are you?"

She laughed. "Let's not have chicken tonight." "Ok," I said, "no chicken."

"Yeah, we've had it too much," she said, and mumbled a few things after. "Are you coming to dinner?" she said.

"Well, no I can't because I have to go home and eat there."

"Ok, sit down, have some milk, maybe some cream," she said as she reached for the table.

"Can I get you something?" I said.

She laughed and said, "Sit down."

I walked closer and said "okay, but would you like some ginger ale?" "Some milk? Why don't we have hot dogs for dinner and we'll have…" she mumbled some other things.

"I can't stay for hot dogs but your dinner will be here soon." "Why can't you stay?"

"I have to go home and eat with my brother."

I didn't know what to say but we've been trained at hospice to follow the conversation if this happens.

"Yeah, your daughter, I mean granddaughter is dating someone so you better go."

I smiled and told her I'd see her soon. Her slipper had fallen off so I went to put it back on but she shook her head no so I took the other one off too and she smiled. I touched her foot to say goodbye and she looked startled and stared at where I touched her sock for a minute. I said bye again, she looked up, said bye and laughed.

Room 223 and 225 were sleeping so I wheeled the cart back to its place, walked across the black asphalt parking lot to chart each patient in the white binder. I left hospice at 18:45 that Friday night and drove out on Ellis Lane with my window down. As I headed west on the interstate, one thing was very clear: it was time for me to leave the field.

The next chapter is a first attempt at understanding the messiness of death and the ways we use language to control and bring order to an otherwise disorderly experience.

· 3 ·

THE MANY WAYS WE USE LANGUAGE

Discourses influence the way we understand life and death. For me, a particular discourse, like a particular model of care, orients us to the world a particular way. Even more, a discourse of care, like emergency medicine or hospice care, for instance, gives us a way of understanding and a way of feeling about death. A particular language influences what we value and what we take to be true, right, and worthy of pursuit. Therefore, to say that there are multiple or competing discourses of care is to say that there are competing ways of understanding life and death, arising with different vocabularies, different ways of interacting, and of making decisions. The more interesting thing is how each discourse and way of understanding life and death is produced, reproduced, and maintained.

By focusing on how discourses orient us to understand life and death in a particular way I have been most interested in language and the way we all use certain vocabularies to achieve certain ends and make distinctions over others. Therefore, I take language seriously and have gained insight from Watson (2003), who underscores that language is not just a tool we use to describe actions; rather, when we speak, we also act. Even more, we bring things into being in large part through the language that we use—and don't use. And when we speak, our words put boundaries around meanings. For example, the words used to describe diagnosis, treatment, and remission have set distinctions around what an illness is and is not.

People "battle" cancer. People "lose" their "fight" with cancer. People "win" their "war" with cancer and become "survivors" with an "army" of support. When we declare "war" on something, we justify the use of an abundance of resources, no matter the emotional, physical, and financial cost. Furthermore, people "kick cancer's ass." Some people "lose" their hair, "lose" their skin color, "lose" their ability to taste and even feel after being lined up like cattle to receive "treatment," and become "cured." People become known as "cancer patients" rather than people with cancer. And we have "cancer centers" rather than "healing centers." These are some of the discourses that have gained considerable momentum through the words and language the members of the medical community, lay people, and the media use over and over. In order to understand the dynamics of language and talk around medical care, I am borrowing insight from a set of literatures whose careful analysis of thinking about discourse and language informs this book.

Like many communication scholars, I believe that language is constitutive. Therefore, organizations like the ED and hospice are discursive constructions because discourse is the very foundation upon which organizational life is built (Fairhurst & Putnam, 2004). The term discourse, however, has a variety of meanings. For me, discourses are broad and general systems of thought that carry values, beliefs, and ideas while encouraging us to think in some ways and not others. They even encourage us to hear in certain ways too, and actively not hear in other ways. What is more, discourses organize and naturalize the world in particular ways, especially around the end of life.

Because language is vital to understanding the relationships between discourse, organizing, and care, it is important to understand how dominant cultural discourses like those about death encourage and constrain the language available to use. For example, a cultural discourse in hospice orients many of us into believing that their care is endlessly different from what we would experience in another setting. This orientation is organized discursively (Broadfoot, 2003; Deetz & Radford, 2008). In general talk, literature, and, as we will see, in providers' language from both sites, hospice is presented as being different from any other place. This presentation is spoken, written, mediated, and unmediated (Foucault, 1973).

In essence, a discourse is a set of interconnected concepts, expressions, and statements that constitute a way of talking and writing about end of life, thereby framing and influencing how people understand and act with regard to care-giving. Discourses distribute meanings around life and death. They also confirm what can be said about death and what should be concealed about death (Broadfoot, 2003). Understanding a discourse includes identifying how language is used in making distinctions between what is a good death, what is a right way to die, and what is worthy in the pursuit of living and dying. It also includes identifying what and whose values and interests are carried with those distinctions in coordinating decisions around end of life (Deetz, 1992).

Broadfoot's (2003) study of a genetic clinic eloquently shows how language coordinates decisions within clinical settings. In her study, she described the meeting that took place when parents sat down with doctors and clinical providers to discuss treatment options for their child with a genetically-based disorder. Three different discursive formations surfaced in their talk, organizing knowledge, concepts of a person, and notions of how life and death work. In her observations, each used the discursive formation they drew from as the way the world was when they were receiving care. Therefore, the focus is on the micro-practices by which persons, knowledge, and collective decisions are produced in particular moments, and how discursive formations organize meanings, create distinctions, and provide scripts for behavior, thereby excluding, denying, or marginalizing others (Broadfoot, 2003; Deetz & Radford, 2008).

How we live, breathe, act, and talk depends on existing discourses, our access to them, and the interests they represent (Broadfoot, 2003; Weedon, 1997). To understand, imagine a meditation room full of meditators and meditating bodies. For the most part, the image is quiet and free from any movement or gestures. Occasionally, however, someone will clear their throat, cough, or adjust their pillow or mat. Often, one movement will trigger another movement. According to Pagis (2010), this orchestra of sound and movement merely reflects human nature and human sociality—we tend to react to others, even when surrounded by silence. This same orchestra of sound and movement can be seen in other public places: the classroom, the church, the hospital, and so on.

How do you feel when you walk into a hospital or hospice? How do you walk? Do you talk? What does it sound like? How do you act? What do you smell? What do you hear? Do you follow a set of built-in rules and norms when you enter a hospital or hospice? Without a doubt, these places influence our interaction. Likewise, our actions influence. In doing so, we actively read silence, gestures and breath as we would read speech, turning silence into a form of communication (Pagis, 2010).

As silence becomes something to be read, we simultaneously sort through multiple discourses as they enter our thoughts. During this sorting, our thoughts must connect and coordinate with others in order to make sense. According to Broadfoot (2003):

> A discursive formation or form of rationality or consciousness is a coordinated ensemble of diverse and often oppositional entities, that once disarticulated, lose their synchronicity. When discourses are articulated as a group, they form statements and conceptual figurations (discursive formations), sets of anonymous rules and structural principles (discursive practices), complex interrelations across sites (discursive fields) and when joined by the non-discursive (discursive apparatus), discourses produce objects, subjects and relationships, deploying power and shaping historically specific meanings…and coherence that appears in such a discursive formation is then dependent on the regular dispersion of these individual discourses in multiple institutions, material practices and subjects (p. 42).

Therefore, discourses that we adopt can affect what we believe and how we feel about life and death.

And discourses around end of life take many formations. Settings like an ED and a hospice are comprised of deeper meanings of speech that determine what can be said and what cannot be said. Discourse, like disease, binds and orders truth and time. As Foucault (1973) argues,

> The order of disease is simply a 'carbon copy' of the world of life; the same structures govern each, the same forms of division, the same ordering. The rationality of life is identical with the rationality of that which threatens it (p. 7).

Even more, Foucault (1973) explains that we are dealing with systems that are both natural and ideal: "Natural, because it is in them that diseases state their essential truths; ideal insofar as they are never experienced unchanged and undisturbed" (p. 8). Therefore, in the rational space of disease, discourses occupy a unique role that is hardly avoidable and endlessly neutralizing and ordering the essences of the disease process (Foucault, 1973).

Discourses are pervasive, ubiquitous, and are exercised through multiple and strategic relations that are filled with tension (Foucault, 1976). For Foucault, "discourse is a way of constituting knowledge, it constitutes the nature of the body, conscious and unconscious mind and the emotional life of the subjects it seeks to govern" (Weedon, 1997, p. 104). This governing is exercised rather than possessed, producing relations based on knowledge, relations about how the world works, and relations about the meaning of life and death (Broadfoot, 2003). These relations, however, unfold through our specific ways of knowing about death and dying and our access to them.

Spending time at the ED and hospice helped me understand what people believe about death and dying based on the language that is available to express their meanings and interpret those of others.

I heard firsthand how language makes certain decisions about end of life care possible at the expense of others. The hospice and the ED are unique insofar as their histories and meanings shape a particular way of talking about medicine and care. Therefore, I want to describe a history of each site to illustrate the dynamic relationship between the environment and the language embedded in it.

The History of Emergency Medicine

The demand for emergency services has been an integral feature of modern health care in the United States and other nations. Despite all the attention on providing health care to Americans, EDs continue to serve as the health care safety net for up to 15 percent of the population (Zink, 2006). It is important to note that I have chosen the term "ED" rather than the routine "ER" for a few reasons. First, many emergency physicians feel that the term emergency room is outdated and doesn't accurately portray the organization of care that is delivered by a orchestrated and multilayered department, rather than a single room, especially after 1961, when full-time emergency physicians began practice (Zink, 2006). However, ER is still accurate for small rural environments.

Emergency medicine has always been about the patients. While all specialties in medicine can claim to have patients as their focus, only one has emerged to take care of anyone, with anything, at any time, at whatever cost. Emergency medicine came about differently from traditional medical specialties (Zink, 2006). It was fueled by new social and political conditions and responded to specific needs of the unwell and the poor, regardless of race.

One particular way health care changed post–World War II was an infu-sion of public reliance on hospital emergency rooms (Zink, 2006). As patients began to seek out care in ERs in the 1950s, the medical expertise for providing quality emergency care was lacking. Specifically,

> Medicine was put into a position of having to catch up to the public demand, but the professional solution to the ER problem did not arise until the 1960s. Some of the physicians who would provide the solution and would later have significant roles in the founding of emergency medicine were in their formative years or were starting their careers in the 1950s. (Zink, 2006, p. 2)

General practitioners and house calls also gave way to emergency care, which slowly subverted the ER into an alternative, costly, primary care setting. Many younger physicians at this time were making fewer house calls and sending more patients to their offices or the hospital, places that had better equipment for a proper exam, and better resources for treatment and diagnosis (Zink, 2006).

The post-World War II era brought increased business and increased in-comes to physicians. In doing so, it also created a community that was fasci-nated with the physician as a professional, scientist, god-like healer. But as patient admissions increased, the ER was generally viewed as an annoyance rather than an opportunity for medical care.

From 1965 to 1970, ED visits in the U.S. rose from 29 million to 42 mil-lion per year, in part because of the increase in Medicare and Medicaid (Zink, 2006). In the mid-1960s, the poor and elderly viewed the hospital as a place where medical care was based, especially in the U.S. Specifically,

> Hospitals had become little fiefdoms of health care in most communities, with out-patient clinics and private physician office buildings adjacent or annexed to the hos-pital building. For patients who were now entitled to care by way of having Medicare and Medicaid insurance, presenting to the ED at a hospital complex was the simplest and most convenient way to gain entry in to a system that could seem imposing and confusing from the outside. Patients understood that even if their problems were not very acute or severe, they would be seen and treated in the ED and referred to outpa-tient care in the same system. Even patients with a regular doctor used the ED in the evening and night hours when accessing their physician was becoming increasingly difficult. (Zink, 2006, p. 56)

Emergency medicine grew up at a time when American medicine was becom-ing more "corporate." The increase in hospitals, insurance companies, and medical specialists in line with the vast amount of money spent meant that health care would become a major industry.

With the continuous changes in medical health care, increases in Medicare, health maintenance organizations (HMOs), and primary care physicians, ED visits should have decreased. However, this has not been the case. Arguably, the most consistent aspect of health care in the past 30 years is ED patient visits (Zink, 2006). Specifically, U.S. ED patient visits were 81 million in 1980, 96 million in 1992, and 114 million in 2002 (American Hospital Association, 1974–2002).

Many believe one factor that has contributed to the increasingly high admission rates to the ED is the passage of the federal Emergency Treatment and Labor Act (EMTALA) in 1986. This piece of legislation was

> Intended to outlaw the practice of patient dumping from one hospital to another. As the healthcare marketplace struggled in the 1980s, some hospitals refused to accept, or inappropriately transferred indigent or uninsured patients to other hospitals— usually to municipal or charity hospitals. A few highly publicized bad outcomes from this practice prompted Congress to act. EMTALA mandated that all hospitals participating in the Medicare program must provide an ED screening evaluation and stabilization or arrange an appropriate transfer without consideration for the patient's ability to pay. (Zink, 2006, p. 274)

Interestingly, after EMTALA, visits to the ED accelerated. Additionally, the overcrowding of waiting rooms was increased by the closure of hundreds of mostly smaller U.S. hospitals and emergency departments in the 1990s. Further, the increase in ED admissions as well as the overcrowding of waiting rooms occurred simultaneously with an increase in the estimated 45 million people who had no insurance.

ED visits for critically ill patients increase as the population ages and sicker people are treated outside of the hospital, despite many assumptions that the increase in admission is a result of "non-acute" or minor illnesses. But since the 1950s, "patients have figured out where they can and in some cases, must go when the health care system cannot provide timely care. People vote with their feet, and the steady march of patients to EDs in the U.S. and worldwide over recent decades suggests that emergency physicians are providing something that is lacking elsewhere in medicine" (Zink, 2006, p. 275).

Because so many people over-rely on them, EDs are viewed by many as a significant contributor to the outrageous health care costs. Others believe if only we could get the people out of the ED who don't belong there, we could bring costs under control. Arguments abound. But despite which argument you choose, the demand for emergency services is remarkable and has been a dominant trend of modern health care, thereby changing the way emergency medicine is practiced and the way it manages its care environment. Many argue that the expertise of emergency physicians has increased more than in any field of medicine. This is a field and a place so many of us turn to in a moment of crisis surrounding life, death, or disability, and it is a place whose history reveals much about the role language plays in order to respond to such demands while remaining the only specialty to take care of anyone, with anything, at any time.

ED physicians have standard protocols and conversations when patients arrive. Here is one example of clinical interaction in the ED I witnessed was when I was shadowing Dr. Mead:

"I'm Dr. Mead and this is Carey, one of our student observers. What's going on that brought you into the hospital?"

"I fell down some stairs and my neck hurts, and I have a bad headache."

"How did you fall?"

"I was wearing flip flops."

"Where does it hurt?"

"Right here" [touches the back of her neck and head].

"When'd you fall?"

"A few hours ago."

"Any previous medical history?"

"Depression" [keeps touching her neck]. Doc walks closer and looks in her ears and then puts pressure on her neck, asking where it hurts. He touches her actual body for about a minute.

"I'd like to get a Catscan and X ray of your neck and head to make sure there is nothing else there."

"Do I have to go in a tube, because I am claustrophobic?"

"You'll be all right. Do you need anything for pain—ibuprofen, something stronger?"

"Something stronger."

"Vicodin? Percocet?"

"Vicodin hurts my stomach."

"Well let's try Percocet. Ok, I will be back in to tell you the results when we have them."

This standard form of interaction—albeit with different details—is known as a clinical algorithm (Groopman, 2007). The patient presents her story and the physician translates her story into an actionable list to reach a therapy or diagnosis. In this case, the patient's story describing pain in the back of her neck from falling is interpreted into action. Following a series of standard questioning and answering, this action translates to ordering a Catscan and X ray of her head and neck.

According to Groopman's (2007) book, *How Doctors Think*, the trunk of the clinical decision tree consists of a patient's major symptoms or laboratory results, contained within a box. Arrows branch from the first box to other boxes. For example, a common symptom like "sore throat" would begin the algorithm, followed by a series of branches with "yes" or "no" questions about associated symptoms. Is there a fever or not? Are swollen lymph nodes associated with the sore throat? Have family members suffered from this symptom? Similarly, a laboratory test like a throat culture for bacteria would appear farther down the trunk of the tree, with branches based on "yes" or "no" answers to the results of the culture. Ultimately, following the branches to the end should lead to the correct diagnosis and therapy (Groopman, 2007).

Clinical algorithms may be useful for run-of-the-mill diagnoses and treatments, but they quickly fall apart when a doctor needs to think outside their algorithmic boxes, when symptoms are vague, or multiple and confusing, or when test results are inexact. In such cases—the kinds of cases where we most need a discerning doctor—algorithms discourage physicians from thinking independently and creatively. Instead of expanding a doctor's thinking, they constrain it. And how should doctors think in clinical settings to account for the complexities of disease and the unique circumstances of an individual's life and health?

Medical interactions in a setting like an emergency department constitute a significant part of the day-to-day practice of clinical medicine (Mishler, 1984). Therefore, talk in this setting has been understood in the literature as a primary source of understanding clinical work. Whose interests does their talk serve? How does it shape and organize the medical encounter as a particular type of language? What type of relationship between patient and physician does it affirm? These questions grow out of a concern as to whether current forms of clinical practice respect the dignity of patients as persons and support recognition of their problems within the context of their lifeworlds or meaning (Mishler, 1984). Drawing from this literature, the groups for interpretation shift from assumptions based on a biomedical model by physicians to the perspective of patients and the lifeworld context of their problems. Therefore, this approach views language seriously—it is not mere talk, but the work that doctor, nurse, and patient do together that is an essential and critical component of clinical practice (Mishler, 1984). This particular understanding of what the patient means in medical interactions tends to be defined as technical, regardless of whether evidence-based medicine or clinical algorithms are in play (Mishler, 1984).

From these perspectives, laboratory tests and the results of physical examinations take priority over what can be learned from talking with patients. The impact of a biomedical model on clinical training, however, is profound. Arguably, hospitals in general, and emergency departments in particular, are the primary settings within which medical students, interns, and residents see patients, yet they have little opportunity to work with patients in the context of general medical practice, as in a primary care setting (Groopman, 2007). Although diagnosis, care, and treatment in these settings are short term, they can be the most important hours for the patients. Even more, they often focus on single episodes of illness in patients who students are unlikely to see again. Thus, talk and training here differ in significant ways from talk and training in other settings such as a primary care or a hospice setting (although this is changing), where physicians and nurses are believed to enter into long term relationships with patients whose life circumstances they become familiar with as they attend to a variety of episodes and illnesses over an extended period of time (Mishler, 1984).

A diagnosis, as described in the literature, is a way of interpreting and organizing observations. According to Mishler (1984), a diagnosis is no less real because it is dependent on what physicians ask and what they hear, and on what patients report and do not report, than it would be if it were based on the results of physical examinations and laboratory tests. Since the discovered illness is constructed and not found, it is, in this sense, partly a function of the talk between a patient and a physician. Thus, the study of talk is central to an understanding of both illness and the meanings of life and death. How end-of-life communication produces and reproduces knowledge about particular medical conditions; how patients see and describe their illness; how providers describe and narrate their cases to their medical colleagues; how providers seek to persuade one another about diagnoses and clinical management, and how they justify and legitimate their knowledge and opinions are central to this project (Mishler, 1984; Foster, 2007). Emergency medicine, therefore, is a communicative activity (Eisenberg et al., 2005).

Unlike other areas of the hospital, the ED is unbounded, meaning that medical practitioners' workloads, patient admissions, flow of work pace, and work environment are essentially uncontrollable. Moreover, the demands on emergency services are increasing during an exceptional time with a provider shortage, rising insurance rates, and more uninsured individuals, thereby implying a new environment for providers, patients, and families (Eisenberg et al., 2005). For that reason, emergency work involves multiplicity, caring for numerous patients with highly variable complaints simultaneously.

The high level of uncertainty that characterizes ED work—in the lack of background information about patients and the need to make difficult decisions before receiving critical data—demands a continuous shifting of framing and communicating. Furthermore, ED work is provided under significant time constraints with stringent charting practices, which can cause a narrowing of focus and a rush to judgment (Eisenberg et al., 2005). Additionally, the lack of long-term relationships with patients leads ED staff to receive little or no feedback about the results of their care, making it difficult to learn from experience. In other words, there is little opportunity for reflective practice (Schön, 1983). Much of ED work is routine, and the riskiest procedures are done only sporadically, in contrast to other specialists, such as surgeons or cardiologists, who perform the riskiest maneuvers up to several times a day (Eisenberg et al., 2005). Together, these norms reveal emergency work to be an important environment in which to study communication and its impact on important health outcomes like end-of-life care.

Unlike most other industries today, health care remains highly fragmented by discipline and function (Schön, 1983). This fragmentation penetrates deeply into healthcare organizations and presents challenges for effective cross-functional communication. For example, EDs are separated by discipline and function, producing significant obstacles to effective communication. Consequently, talk in EDs is internally fragmented by professional barriers separating physicians from nurses and nurses from interns, residents, techs, aides, and EMTS, and externally fragmented by the frequent presence and influence of other specialists such as consultants, pre-hospital service providers, laboratory, radiology, and others. Despite years of effort to create effective cross-functional healthcare teams, with some success, they still remain mediocre since most healthcare providers identify more strongly with their particular function or profession (nursing, radiology, cardiology, or pediatrics) than with their home institution or healthcare system (Eisenberg et al., 2005).

Understanding EDs as communication environments directs attention to how interaction processes construct and maintain ED culture, as well as to which patterns of interaction are likely to lead to less effective decisions and medical errors (Eisenberg et al., 2005). A significant element of such an analysis focuses on the politics of participation in decision-making, that is, how certain interests, values, and rationalities take precedence over others.

A useful conceptualization for understanding the basic forms of rationality within emergency medicine is Browning's (1992) discussion of lists and stories as forms of organizational talk. According to Browning, two forms of rationality operate in every institution. The first, technical rationality, involves classification and developing lists. Scripts, lists, algorithms, checklists, and formal processes are all ways of encoding the technical knowledge used by individuals in their work. And in any organization, much of the work consists of the enactment and execution of agreed-upon lists or routines—ways of planning, organizing, designing, or producing a particular product or service, like delivering care.

A second kind of rationality is narrative, expressed in the stories people tell. Many organizational activities rely on storytelling, from new employee socialization, to medical training and education, to organizational planning. In healthcare settings like an emergency department, patients arrive with a story, and a significant component of medical training focuses on how to create a supportive environment wherein patients will feel comfortable to tell their story (Charon, 2006). Creating this type of environment, however, is more complex than a simple shifting from list to story. In fact, much of the literature describes talk and language as too "easy" or straightforward in an environment that is inherently complex, dynamic, and fluid. The complexity of talk beyond technical or narrative rationality is visible even in triage encounters, like the one I observed below between a nurse, a patient, and the patient's father. Again, I recorded this interaction on a scratch piece of paper and therefore have not cleaned up—or changed—any words or phrases.

Nurse:	Hi, what's going on?
Dad:	Well we are getting frequent flyers to the ER!
[Laughter]	
Patient:	I've had a terrible pain in my stomach and the past five times I've been here they have told me it is appendicitis.
Nurse:	Do you have your appendix?
Patient:	Yes.
Nurse:	Does anything you do make it worse or better?
Patient:	No.
Nurse:	How long has the pain been going on?
Patient:	A few weeks.
Nurse:	Okay Dad, I need you to step out while I ask her a couple questions.

Dad: OK.
Nurse: Alright sister, anything I need to know?
Patient: No.
Nurse: Any chance you are pregnant?
Patient: No!
Nurse: Are you sexually active?
Patient: No.
Nurse: Do you do drugs?
Patient: Well, yeah.
Nurse: Which ones?
Patient: Well, I do, I have smoked weed.
Nurse: Okay, how often?
Patient: Like two months and again like two weeks ago.
Nurse: Okay, that's not good for you, you know? Anything else?
Patient: No.
Nurse: Okay, I'll get your dad and we'll go back.
Dad: Now do you need me again to talk about insurance?
[Laughter and they walk back]

Talk in the ED, as this example illustrates, is not easily classified into stories and lists. Talk in this setting is candid, emotional, performative, and unpredictable. Even more, talk must endlessly be understood in a way that reflects a person's lived experience, not just their medical experience (Charon, 2006; Schön, 1983). Recent work in medical education, however, focuses specifically on the critical role of narrative rationality in effective patient care (Charon, 2006; Eisenberg et al., 2005). Therefore, the relevance of Browning's (1992) conception of the study of emergency medicine has to do with the continual interplay between these two competing forms of rationality. Patients and families come to the ED with stories, and the institutional response is to seek to translate their stories into actionable lists. Browning (1992) elaborates:

> The list is rooted in science and presented in a formula for action leading to controllable outcomes. The list represents standards, accountability, certainty, and reportability. Conversely, the story is romantic, humorous, conflicted, tragic and most of all, dramatic...stories fill the breaks in technical rationality. Narrative rationality fills the loose coupling between intentions and outcomes. (pp. 281–282)

The movement from story to list can be smooth, particularly when the patient reports routine or standard symptoms on what appears to be a direct disease process.

Doctors learn about diagnosis early on in medical school, which employs technical rationality to match patients' complaints to specific diagnostic categories (Charon, 2006). Patients whose symptoms are vague, ambiguous, and suggest multiple conflicting diagnoses do not have a "good" story. And extreme pressures on time and space do not provide a supportive environment for the deliberate interpretation of patient narratives (Eisenberg et al., 2005). Instead, the care team makes the best decision possible, whether it is ordering more tests, collecting more data, or discharging the patient. These, in turn, transition into action, following the list that seems most useful (i.e., lab tests, diagnosis, treatments).

ED physicians routinely characterize patients who report clear, recognizable symptoms as having a "good story," meaning that there is a simple and specific translation to an actionable list that at the same time rules out alternative diagnoses. Stories are used throughout a patient's stay. For example, at the end of a patient's stay, some degree of translation from list to story is always necessary. Essentially, there are three ways to leave the ED: discharge, hospital admission, or death—each type of exit requiring a story. Discharge requires some form of treatment plan, while hospital admission requires the team to persuade the patient that their condition is severe enough to be admitted to the hospital. And a patient's death requires the care team to develop a convincing story to assure family and friends that they did all they could for their loved one. Thus, communication side-steps a thin line stretching from the meaning of technical results and procedures on the one hand to the complexity of the patient's condition on the other (Eisenberg et al., 2005).

Emergency providers are the ones we go to when we can't see our regular doctor, don't have insurance, get sick in the middle of the night, are in an accident, stub our toe, can't breathe well, don't know how to care for someone, or don't have someone to care for us. In essence, we ask much of this profession and this form of care, whose history is as rich and complex as the language used for providing the care. It is a specialty whose meaning is as unique and diverse as the services it offers to anyone. Dr. Brian Keaton, a past president of the American College of Emergency Physicians (ACEP), specifically articulates the profession and meaning of emergency medicine as the following:

> Patients have spoken with their feet, seeking emergency department care in unprecedented numbers. We are the ones you come to when you're really sick, possibly sick, or kind of sick and in need of rapid evaluation, diagnosis, and treatment. We are the place you come to when you cannot or will not wait for others to find a place in their schedules for you, and the site of medical refuge when you don't know where else to turn. Despite limited resources, unrealistic expectations, and impossible demand,

emergency medicine delivers on our promise to provide the best possible care to every patient regardless of their ability to pay or what time of day they choose to seek care. Alan Kay once said, "the best way to predict the future is to invent it." We're in an inventing mode and are being presented with a historic opportunity to define the future of our specialty and of American medicine. The opportunities in emergency medicine are endless and by choosing this career you will become a leader and a champion for the health care needs of your patients. The challenges before our health care system and emergency medicine are significant, but the rewards and honor of providing care to our communities are limitless. (Keaton, 2007, pp. 5–6)

Thus, the meaning of emergency medicine expands beyond the studies or ideas about medical talk described earlier. Furthermore, while claiming that talk is curative and translating things into clinical representation may be accurate, it is grossly oversimplified. Understanding the competing discourses of care around end of life is very different, in the ED, from translating between list and stories. Relieving patients' suffering is a goal of both emergency medicine and hospice medicine. Although their concerns may be the same, their language, context, and purpose in relieving a patient's suffering are different.

The History of Hospice Care

Hospice care is as complex and critical as emergency care. Hospice care dates back to the 6th and 7th centuries, with the spread of Christianity in Europe. Though end-of-life care was provided at home, many monasteries accepted sick and dying people who did not have family to care for them (Ragan et al., 2008). This type of care for the dying provided at the monasteries continued throughout the Middle Ages and the Crusades, and well into the 17th century, as people who were ill and dying often spent their last days being cared for by monks, nurses, and lay women (Ragan et al., 2008). As the field of medicine began to evolve and formal hospitals were established, people who were ill and dying were treated and cared for in hospitals.

Care for people who were dying, provided through the services of the church, shifted to institutionalized care in hospitals. Unfortunately, early hospital environments did not know enough to guard against germs and disease, which often meant that hospitalized individuals contracted and died from diseases other than those for which they were admitted (Ragan et al., 2008). As a result, early hospitals earned a poor reputation and were viewed as death houses. Under this circumstance, early end-of-life care shifted again to home care provided by family members and neighbors. Care continued at home despite advances in medicine and the established effectiveness of hospitals after World War II. As the knowledge of germ theory and the origins of disease were developed, medical treatments expanded, and the focal point of health care turned exclusively to saving lives and curing diseases. Individuals who were dying were seen as medical failures because their cases could not advance medical knowledge (Ragan et al., 2008). In short, care for the dying was not considered within the scope of medicine.

The term hospice is of Latin origin, "hospes," meaning to be a guest or stranger. The term was first used by Madame Jeanne Gernier, who founded the Dames de Calaire in Lyon, France in 1842. In 1879, the Irish Sisters of Charity opened Our Lady's Hospice in Dublin, Ireland. Mother Teresa, known as one of the founders of hospice care, opened the Kalighat Home for the Dying in 1952. Dame Cicely Saunders started the first hospice program at St. Christopher's in London in 1967. The religious roots of hospice care facilitated the growth of the movement and formalized care of the dying as hospice care. The movement spread, and the first hospice program in North America was established in 1974 in New Haven, Connecticut (Ragan et al., 2008).

Patients' experiences led to the opening of the first modern research and teaching hospice, St. Christopher's, in London in 1967. Saunders (2003), the founder of the hospice, writes,

> While working at St. Joseph's Hospice in East London with the Irish Sisters of Charity, where I spent seven years on an extensive study on *The Nature and Management of Terminal Pain* (Saunders, 1967), I began making tape recordings of many of my patients...As I wrote then and many times since, what was being talked about was "total pain"—"all of me is wrong." Without any further questioning [other than 'tell me about your pain'] she had talked of her mental as well as her physical distress, of her social problems and of her spiritual need for security. Then, as now, I know that listening to a patient's own tale of their troubles can be therapeutic in itself. As another patient said, "it seemed the pain went with me talking." (pp. 4–6)

Therefore, it was the intentional listening to suffering patients' voices that inspired the opening of the first real hospice, in 1967. Similarly, this intentional listening to suffering patients has served as endless inspiration for this study.

The medicalization of grief and bereavement that occurred during the 1950s gained momentum, as death began to occur less at the home and more at the hospital. According to Littlewood (1993), the medical community believed it was its responsibility to keep death away from the community. Yet little attention was paid to the dying process, and little care was given to those who were terminally ill (Ragan et al., 2008). Hospice is a care service that excludes curative treatment of illness, opting for holistic care of terminally ill patients. The primary goal in hospice care is pain and symptom management at the end of the disease progression. And the paramount goal of hospice care, particularly out-patient, is to provide patients with the opportunity to die at home, surrounded by loved ones, with as little pain as possible (Ragan et al., 2008).

Hospice provides a team approach to medical care, pain management, and emotional and spiritual support in order to individualize care for the person and their family's needs and wishes. In order to be eligible for hospice care, the patient's doctor and the hospice medical director use their best clinical judgment to certify that the patient is terminally ill, with life expectancy of six months or less, if the disease runs its standard course. Hospice care focuses on the belief that every individual has the right to die pain-free and with dignity, and that loved ones will receive the support to allow this to happen. For that reason, hospice is an inherently communicative environment that creates and maintains relationships through communication about the meanings surrounding life and death.

Making communication profound in hospice care is how people are together near the end of someone's life; they create a new relationship at a time when life consists mostly of loss. And these relationships are often filled with intimacy and immediacy. Foster (2007), who worked ethnographically as a volunteer at hospice, discusses how patients did not care about her level of education, what she did for a living, or where she was from. What ultimately mattered in her relationship with patients was the kind of person she was, the interests she showed in patients, and her commitment to being there to share their life. It is about allowing the relationship and communication to reveal itself, learning to improvise and respond spontaneously to each other in the moment (Foster, 2007).

Improvising communication and care and building relationships during a time when life is ending are unique, as Western thinking about death centers around individuals' understanding of self (Walter, 1994). When I started noticing the extraordinary forms of loss that occur at the end of life, I remember having coffee with a friend and colleague, asking her what happens when everything you've known, said, read, taught, touched, felt, loved, and feared, goes away and means nothing to anyone else? What is left of us? She smiled and touched her heart and said, "just this, just this." And what is the meaning of all that stuff when it loses its significance? She smiled again and said, "makes you think, doesn't it?" The relationship between hospice workers and patients calls into question the standard paradigm of autonomy and control that many of us are used to having (Foster, 2007). The relational communication of the mundane, the moments, the silences, and the whispers distinguish hospice as a human and comforting alternative conception of dying.

Communication in hospice occurs in the silences and simple activities of life. It fosters listening over judging or imposing values onto patients and their families. Improvisation overrules agenda-setting. The implicit principle that centers on the patient's needs adapts communication to the patient's worldview and preferences (Foster, 2007).

Many believe the contexts in which care is delivered and the barriers to "good" care contrast starkly with that of a clinical or curative setting. But how, in practice, do providers listen to each and every individual passing through a palliative care unit, in-patient hospice, out-patient hospice, or bereavement agency? Can systems of care actually be developed for something so personal as the end of life? Can death really be tailored according to personal preference? Would we want that anyway? Can our old—and often standard—models of funerals represent the complexity and extraordinary nature of human life (Walter, 1994)?

These questions matter for a philosophy of care whose primary goal is treating each person as an individual and respecting the feelings, beliefs, and wishes of the dying person. Dame Cicely Saunders envisioned the communication between hospice workers and families as one of dialogue, an explicitly "I and thou" relationship (Bradshaw, 1996; Buber, 1958; Foster, 2007). Buber himself argued that true dialogue is limited within an unequal "helping" relationship, such as the volunteer-patient relationship, and tends to be minimal when it does occur (Foster, 2007). This conception of communication has been used to describe how language shapes relationships at hospice through specific interaction processes.

Dialogue is relational and responsive, and an interaction process that underscores how talk is an essential building block of community at a place like hospice (Foster, 2007; Buber, 1958). Buber's philosophy of dialogue depends on how the self interprets the other, or "thou." Buber is not suggesting by "thou-ness" that every relationship should move toward intimacy and the disclosure/realization of the other's real self, but that the "realness" of the other resists fixed meaning or a closure of conversation. Every interaction holds the possibility of closure or new meaning. Dialogue is a process used to explain how patients, families, volunteers, and providers engage differently around end of life (Foster, 2007). And in so doing, communication becomes productive, creating something new together as opposed to reproducing what either individual has or is.

The ability, then, to achieve the ideals of dialogue is both facilitated and complicated by the practice of multidisciplinary teamwork in hospice consisting of nurses, physicians, case workers, dietitians, chaplains, and bereavement and activity counselors, who all inform and influence care team goals and decisions.

Seale (1998) identified the emergence of dialogue as part of a larger movement toward patient-centered medicine and away from clinical medicine, which had made the voice of the patient less relevant. Achieving this form of communication, however, requires responsibility, responsiveness, and accountability. Improvisation, for example—something that is embraced—demands a high degree of skill and familiarity with the context and the role one is playing, and enough confidence to surrender to the moment (Eisenberg, 1990; Weick, 1998). One study, for instance, about active listening was ranked as the most frequently implemented nursing intervention used to "enhance and support the spirituality of clients and their families" around hospice care (Sellers & Haag, 1998, pp. 347–348). This model of communication, however, is both difficult to implement into practice and has received its own critiques, as Walter (1994) states rather poignantly:

> On the one hand, they [hospice workers] are committed to letting patients live as they wish until they die. On the other hand, hospices have a very clear idea of 'the good death'….These are the two classic strands that together make a revival: a late-modern/neo-traditional attempt to promote a particular idea of healthy dying, and a postmodern enabling of individuals to do it their own way. (p. 89)

Therefore, a tension arises between encouraging the patients' autonomy and remaining nondirective while advocating a "good death." Even more, providers are encouraged to negotiate between the directives of the organization, the patient's wishes, and their own values. This balance is learned not through intellect, but through experience (Foster, 2007). Hospice workers are not change agents. Rather, they bear witness, support, and comfort the individual and family physically, emotionally, and socially (Foster, 2007).

Hospice care, like emergency care, focuses on language, the body, and negotiating endless tensions and wishes. Human bodies are undeniably mortal and it is the symbolic constructions, the words, that ward off senses of mortality and extend the human body toward life (Becker, 1997). Since language has come to disassociate bodies from mortality, language has also become the power families, patients, and the public turn to at the hour of death and also what providers turn to when coordinating care around the end of life (Foster, 2007). Yet simply focusing on thoughts and words overlooks how our bodies and emotions are also dependent on our access to certain discourses (Seale, 1998).

Caring for bodies and emotions through language, improvisation, and relationships is a central goal of both hospice and palliative medicine. It is about relieving patients' suffering—at the end of life (hospice) and during the entire course of serious, advanced illness (palliative medicine)—while also maintaining quality of life for them (Ragan et al., 2008). The focus is on patients' comfort and physical needs and on their emotional, social, and spiritual needs. The health care approach is patient-centered, as patients are able to dictate what they need and want during both critical illnesses and in their last days or weeks.

Studies of talk and language are where actual and possible forms of organizing are defined and contested. The ways we represent our lived experiences and relationships to ourselves and our existence begin to unfold (Broadfoot, 2003). Understanding talk is also a way of understanding discourses and our access to them—how individuals perceive, think, and talk about emergency departments and hospice.

The histories and experiences of an emergency department and a hospice remind us how much we take for granted, and how much we can be moved by the words and stories of others. Even more, these worlds of unique discourses, interconnected concepts, revealing expressions, and stunning statements illustrate how talk subtly frames and influences how people understand and act in the face of life and death.

· 4 ·

SOME THEORIES FOR MAKING SENSE
OF COMMUNICATION AND DYING

Interaction is dynamic. And language, meaning, and experience are at the root of many of the problems faced by dying patients and their families (Hickman, 2002). Other individuals, organizational structures, media, and cultural environments influence us all.

Communication issues are central to discussions about how to improve care for people who are dying. Dying practices can be lonely, mechanical, and impersonal. Contrasted with a romanticized view of loved ones by the bedside, patients are now often surrounded by busy nurses, interns, residents, lab technicians, or researchers who are all strangers, mostly because they discuss the value of life in a language that makes sense in their world, a language often different from that of those who are dying.

Like patients, physicians struggle to balance straightforward communication about terminal illness. They, too, have their own fears of getting sick, or know someone who has been sick. They must also be sensitive to timing, sensitive to patient preferences, and sensitive to the accuracy of their prognoses. Above all, providers are encouraged to offer some kind of hope, even if hope is oriented to maximizing quality of life rather than extending it. (Wenrich et al., 2001). Dying and attending to the death of another person can present communication challenges for everyone involved.

The medical encounter has primarily been studied as an interpersonal communication event (Street, 2003). Specifically, it has focused on patterns of interaction between provider and patient, and the nature of their relationship. Understanding the medical encounter interpersonally means enhancing providers' and patients' ability to make useful and thoughtful communication choices in practical clinical situations. The term "useful" refers to developing choices that enable patients and providers to accomplish their own care goals, as well as create opportunities for future clinical interactions.

Because talk is almost always between a provider and patient or a provider and family, medical talk is an interpersonal activity. Therefore, an interpersonal approach allows me to start thinking about what providers and patients need to know to interact productively, rather than reviewing what we already know. This shift in focus allows us to understand communication more as a process instead of a simple transmission of meaning.

Communication is a process that develops in response to a variety of conflicting goals. Patients and providers enter the medical encounter with specific goals in mind and throughout their interaction are endlessly negotiating these goals, or, literally, working through them together. And clearly, interactions can be of value, meaning that interactions are productive and open, or they can be futile, meaning that interactions are reproductive and closed.

Developing skills for communicating about end of life is nothing new. In fact, the topic has gained considerable attention with the help of the multicenter SUPPORT study (1995). This study demonstrated devastating problems in the care of seriously ill hospitalized patients. Specifically, it revealed that only 47% of physicians knew when their patients preferred do-not-resuscitate status. Also, this study illustrates how communicating preferences regarding resuscitation is a challenging and important task for physicians (Chittenden, Clark & Pantilat, 2006).

Understanding patients' wishes at the end of life allows clinicians to prevent unwanted interventions, and to promote dignity and autonomy among patients (Chittenden et al., 2006). Because of the dynamics of providers' and patients' interactions, much of the health promotion research has been more focused on developing mass communication–style messages to influence health beliefs and behaviors. But we need more research examining the exchange of interpersonal messages, especially concerning communication at the end of life. Understanding the medical encounter as an interpersonal event moves us beyond simply thinking that the encounter is a face-to-face monologue, to one where there is dialogue, and a genuine effort and curiosity to understand the other through trust and openness.

An Interpersonal Approach

An interpersonal model of communication provides an important perspective on the dimensions of coordinating care around end of life. However, this view of communication often falls victim to many Western world perspectives about human interaction, where communication is understood as the transmission of ideas from a patient (i.e., sender) to a provider (i.e., receiver), or simply as the exchange of messages, or what one person says and the other hears. Unfortunately, this specific understanding of communication often does not serve us very well in a highly mediated, pluralistic, and interdependent world (Deetz & Radford, 2008). Studies that understand the medical encounter as an interpersonal activity often offer a set of skills—in some cases, very good ones—but do not capture the complexities of communication at the end of life. To continue exploring the dynamics and consequences of talk, I have taken a comprehensive approach to examining end-of-life discussions, gaining insight into the ways in which medical encounters are produced, made, and affected by the contexts in which they are situated (Street, 2003).

Gaining insight into the ways providers and patients can interact productively and sensitively is critical. Part of choosing more productive options in interpersonal interactions also means I pay attention to the gaps in current patterns of talk. These spaces and gaps draw attention to the way we form our experiences of life and death. More importantly, shifting focus to these gaps and spaces is a way to begin to understand how meaning is constructed and contested through interaction. Therefore, I have gained significant insight into the ways in which our clinical interactions, and ideas about life and death, are produced and why this understanding matters.

A Social Construction Approach

A social construction approach to communicating about end of life issues provides awareness of more interesting processes of communication today—how social meanings get produced and reproduced through our patterns of interaction. From a social constructionist perspective, I take the idea that no word, action, behavior, or event has meaning without understanding the larger meaning system in which it is placed. For example, the ED has been produced and reproduced through popular television shows. As a result, it is difficult to think of the ED differently from the larger system of chaos and fast tempo. And therefore, death in the ED becomes difficult or even impossible to understand as something other than beeping monitors, a number of people in the room, IVs thrown on the ground, and sheets ripped off the bed in order to save a life.

Believing that no word, action, behavior, or event has meaning without a larger context of meaning underscores the way language about death and dying carries historical and cultural values and perspectives of which we are rarely aware. These values condition us to act in specific ways that influence what we believe to be true about life and death. Our beliefs, in turn, become socially produced and reproduced through our interactions. These interaction patterns become habitual speech patterns without us ever questioning how or why we accepted them.

To say that values and language influence who we are and what we hold to be true, right, and worthy of pursuit, is to say, more academically, that language shapes our reality. The notion of reality as a social construction has infiltrated recent research in the social sciences, where sociologists Berger and Luckmann's (1966) discussions of the concept gained considerable traction. For example, we act on knowledge that we've learned and accepted through things we've read about death and dying, and develop our communication from other scholars' research on death and dying. Other experiences that we learn from TV, songs, or media give us other ways to understand life and death. These accepted forms of knowledge, based on socially constructed meanings, shape our understanding of life and death and thereby influence what we believe in and take to be true and right.

The idea that language shapes reality obviously leads to theories that our understandings and meanings of death are inherently constructed (Charmaz, 1980; Seale, 1998). Specifically, Charmaz (1980) asserts the following:

> Any sociological exploration into the social reality of death must come to grips with values. Whether values are fixed and stable within a group or are open to reinterpretation, they give rise to the construction of the reality of death. Put simply, death does not occur in a vacuum. Rather, it is a dimension of human existence shaped by values. In particular, I submit that values built on the Protestant Ethos still have a pervasive but subtle effect on death and dying although cultural diversity and biographical experience may give rise to other effects. In that sense, values not only

give rise to meanings of death but also to the everyday practices through which death is handled. (p. 12)

My own values about a good life, a good death, and good medical care have shaped, and been shaped by, my own experiences with health and death as well as what I have experienced in the ED and the hospice. Understanding the medical encounter as a social construction, I share a similar commitment to understanding the way discourse and language in medical settings act to perpetuate the interests of some people over others.

Although some human bodily experiences are universal, such as health, pain, and death, social constructionism argues that such experiences are subjective and understood according to the historical and cultural settings in which they take place, such as EDs and hospices. But in these particular settings, understanding how meanings are produced cannot fully be articulated without considering the ways meanings are shaped within distinct cultural contexts (Lupton, 2003). Therefore, I have also gained insight from a critical cultural approach to communication, because examining the cultural dimensions of medicine and talk sheds light on why medicine and death are "characterized by such strong paradoxes, why issues of health and illness are surrounded with controversy, conflict, and emotion" (Lupton, 2003, p. 2).

A Critical Cultural Approach

Another dialogic approach to understanding talk is a critical cultural view, overtly political through its questioning of how economic, material, and historical factors shape a culture's responses to and concepts of health, disease, and treatment decisions (Lupton, 1994; Lupton, 2003). For me, the term culture is not limited to the traditional anthropological definition. Instead, I understand culture as a way of life, including ideas about treatments, beliefs about health and illness, language used to describe the dying process, the institutions we turn to for help, and the structures of our health care system that shape how we think and feel. I also understand culture to be a range of cultural practices, including artistic formations about the body and disease; architecture, including the physical and material spaces of hospitals and hospices; and further yet, our everyday choices and activities that are in line with—and orient us towards—a particular culture.

Moreover, and of particular interest for this project, is the struggle around defining and naming health, illness, and death. This approach to defining and naming is not only a state of physical or emotional being. Instead, it controls the resources we have available to us to sustain and promote life: medicine, treatment, equipment, providers, food, water, shelter, knowledge, and so on. Through the struggle of naming and defining comes tension and conflict over the ways things are. And in a perfect world, this struggle produces choice. That is, the tension inspires a constructive discussion that would not otherwise have taken place.

Of great interest, then, is the way language forms relationships but in doing so, sets distinctions about life, death, and medical care. For example, I have struggled to name health, disease, and death. What is acceptable for me to say? Should I say "passed" around my family, "died" when I am in the ED, and, use a combination of both when I write, so as to not offend my audience? The language we use about death bespeaks a society struggling to figure out what to value. Therefore, the critical cultural approach engages in a struggle to try to develop alternative languages of medical care and death. Doing so requires difference in the way language is used and the relations and distinctions it puts into play for our understanding of life and death.

Instead of focusing on the individual, a critical cultural approach centers on critiquing the social conditions under which individuals act in regard to medical care. A turn to culture exposes the complexities and contradictions of what a culture does or does not do (Treichler, 1990). Specifically, questions of death are significant in a culture, and significant changes in dying patterns often signal broad cultural change. Even more, "whatever else a culture does or does not do, if it wishes to reproduce itself, it must produce new members" (Treichler, 1990, p. 113). This idea sheds light on the intersection between culture and medicine.

I have gained great insight from Treichler (1990), whose account of medicine and the construction of childbirth paints a wonderful example of the intersection between culture and medical discourse. Her study begins with a cultural "crisis." The term "crisis" is used conventionally to mean a turning point in a sequence of events, after which things get better or worse. Further, Treichler illustrates how childbirth patterns—like dying patterns—in the U.S. are disrupted at many levels: legislative battles over who can legally deliver babies, malpractice and other forms of litigation, rising insurance rates and health care costs, lobbying contests, and market competition (Treichler, 1990). She explains that "these disruptions are played out in language, they embody the tensions and contradictions of the health-care system and the culture in which they occur" (Treichler, p. 115).

These tensions also highlight what a culture is trying to value around health. And if a culture does not merely want to reproduce itself, but to change for the better it must teach its members to think, practice, relate, and learn in new ways.

Treichler's study generates a host of questions about childbirth that are equally relevant for death. For example, where should death take place? Who is best qualified to supervise and pronounce someone dead? Who should decide? How should pain be managed? Who should profit from it? How much should death cost? Who should pay? Who should be paid? In a society as pluralistic as our own, positions and meanings should also be as diverse. But for the most part, meanings remain the same and are reproduced through interaction until a crisis arrives, or a "perfect storm." Crises and storms, however, like those surrounding medicine, society, and economics, often offer a turning point where the negotiation of meaning is contested even in subtle ways, thereby calling into question widely accepted practices and assumptions around dying. Even more, "a crisis that continues long enough may at last destabilize established views of reality" (Treichler, 1990, p. 118). I am not arguing that death is in a crisis, however. Rather, and in line with Treichler, I am arguing that the crisis is not about death per se, but the meanings surrounding death that are produced and reproduced through the way we talk and interact.

Again, the core of any crisis is meaning. What does death mean? To whom? And under what circumstances does a given meaning about death come to constitute an official definition of our experience of it? For Treichler (1990), the problem of traditional childbirth is rooted not in "medicalization" but in monopoly: monopoly of professional authority, material resources, and linguistic capital—that is, the power and access to establish and reinforce a particular definition, whether it is over childbirth or death. For example, death in the U.S. often takes place in hospitals because a definition of death as a medical event is so strong that it determines its material location.

Of interest to Treichler (1990) as well as to this project is the way some meanings come to function as official definitions within a culture. Specifically, it is not about which definition is used, but the process by which definitions are constructed, implemented, and reproduced.

Even more, it is quite plausible, in terms of meaning, to say that multiple meanings may co-exist in a culture. But a definition is much less democratic. It sets limits, and determines boundaries. Unlike meanings, which are bound up in what people think and intend, definitions claim to state what *is*. A definition is a meaning that has become "official" and thereby appears to tell us how things are in the real world. (Treichler, 1990, p. xii)

Definitions around death and dying are outcomes of struggles and crises, however. Therefore, they are also unstable, negotiated, and often temporary (Treichler, 1990). Consequently, proposing a more complex understanding of how definitions of death and dying are created matters. This complexity illuminates the ways language shapes our meanings around dying, professionalism in the clinic, economic resources for treatment, and political activism around new measures surrounding health care and dying practices.

Medical definitions, much like any culture's definitions, determine actual practice and structural arrangements, like the physical space of hospitals and hospices, and our access to them. Definitions also determine political and economic policies and practices, including standard protocols, insurance rates, reimbursement, time providers must work, and time spent with patients. Focusing on the construction of definitions as a complex cultural practice, however, seems difficult or out of place in settings that need to rely on facts, standards, protocols, and consistency. For even talking about the construction of language, discourse, and definitions often generates a desire to return to clarity or certainty about what is real. And the real is always linguistic and political, as well. Therefore, a definition is not, as conventional wisdom assumes, the set of necessary and sufficient conditions that constitute a known, fixed starting point for political, economic, and ideological struggles. Rather, a definition represents the outcome of such struggles–an unstable, negotiated, and often quite temporary cultural prescription (Treichler, 1990, p. 120).

People aren't the problem; the way people talk is the problem. This distinction is important for understanding culture and its dynamic and sentimental relationship with medicine and language.

Understanding culture around end-of-life communication includes focusing on discourse and the way that the use of language in medical settings constitutes relationships as well as distinctions about what we as a society value. Therefore, an understanding of language in both written texts and talk is the primary site of struggle over where meaning is produced, how it is produced, and by whom it is produced (Deetz, 1992). Out of the struggles among competing discourses come tension and the resulting choice to repro-duce something we already have, or produce something new and different (Lupton, 1994). Such an approach recognizes the importance of the discur-sive and linguistic processes by which patterns of illness, health, and death are shaped and perpetuated by our very own talk that is endlessly shaped within particular cultural contexts like an ED and a hospice.

Understanding the role of culture in the organization of end-of-life care and construction matters for our ability to question the existence of essential truths. This doesn't mean it is necessary to abolish essential truths about death and dying. Rather, it asserts that "truth" should be considered the product of tension-filled relations and, as such, is never neutral, but always acting in the interests of someone (Deetz, 1992).

Examining discourse within clinical settings has helped me to under-stand how cultural contexts shape our identities, our feelings, and our emo-tions. Because according to a critical cultural approach, these, of course, are largely discursively produced experiences that are incredibly dynamic and complex. Since discourse, language, and meaning are so central to this study, the consequences of the way we talk as well as identifying where we struggle in our talk is central. Therefore, I can take even more insight about the con-sequences of our talk within cultural contexts by borrowing insight from a dialogic perspective, which offers a way to describe the intimate and complex relations between medicine, culture, and discourse. It also gives us a way to describe the ethical questions of how we should behave, who we truly are, and what we should do as individuals, professionals, and institutions around end of life (Broadfoot, 2003).

A Multi-Method Approach

A critical and dialogic perspective has much to offer this study because it exposes the ways discourses are implemented, negotiated, and transformed with health care providers in EDs and hospices, and with patients, families, and friends. In short, this perspective focuses on the way people discursively construct and contest what it means to be healthy or terminally ill in the 21st century.

Critical approaches start with the basic ontology that our perceptions constitute our realities as we attach meaning to experiences and events, and that these meanings arise through interactions (Alvesson & Deetz, 2000). Therefore, they also start with an epistemological assumption that we come to agreement about what is real intersubjectively. An epistemological assumption is concerned with questions about "how do we know, and how can we come to know." For example, different people approach the end of life and make decisions about how they want to die differently. Some may want to have all the facts and data about their disease and want to know exactly how many days they have left to live. But these same people might be moved by a story of someone else's experience with the disease or preference for dying. The story, then, becomes a different way of knowing and a different way of orienting towards end of life.

Therefore, to say that we come to agreement about what is real intersubjectively is similar to the belief that others understand and know what we are going through, and vice versa (Pagis, 2010). In everyday life, and often without recognition, we tend to live a big part of our lives in other people's minds (Pagis, 2010). As a result, we often take on these other ways of knowing as if they were our own, and as if they were our only options. Therefore, a critical approach sheds light on how we often unknowingly accept routine practices, without critical examination, as preferred ways of knowing and thinking. Even more, a critical approach underscores the processes by which we come to agree on a shared experience and a shared feeling, for example, around the end of life.

For this to occur, critical approaches are unique insofar as they challenge dominant discourses, or dominant ways of knowing, in order to get discussions going in places where they may not seem needed (Alvesson & Deetz, 2000). And a place where discussion is often strained or avoided is around death and our preferred ways of dying. Critical approaches help to bring topics like death back into discussion. In doing so, a critical approachs help generate more discussions and thereby includes more voices around end of life. Incorporating more voices matters for developing new understandings rooted in cultures that can define experiences through a vocabulary that they helped to create. Further, this way of interacting acknowledges difference through genuine listening, understanding, and willingness to be changed, especially in interaction with others' experiences, meanings, and languages that are different from ours (Deetz, 1992; Zoller & Kline, 2008). Similarly, this open, communicative attitude is a goal of a dialogic perspective, which helps me further understand the dynamics of talk in the ED and hospice.

A dialogic approach seeks to inspire a discussion where none seems to exist, albeit differently from a critical approach. Specifically, in order to generate more discussions and have different voices included in defining experience around end of life, a dialogic perspective sees interaction as an endless struggle (Alvesson & Deetz, 2000). Even more, a dialogic perspective helps me to see interaction as a site of struggle between diverse forms of knowing, being, and speaking in the ED and hospice. In so doing, it helps expose the multiple ways people discursively construct and understand death and dying as things are endlessly experienced through interaction.

Importantly, this model of interaction matters around end-of-life communication because within struggle, particular perspectives and voices are often suppressed in order to stabilize and provide shared meaning for participants. For example, if someone says they are not afraid to die, we often always assume they must be "death-denying," since their story and perspective are essentially re-writing the meaning of end-of-life. For understanding end-of-life communication, the critical evaluation of these moments of struggle matters because these are the moments where individuals attempt to make sense of coherent worlds out of hidden and fragmented points of discursive struggle. For example, when I first started observing hospice, the nurse practitioner told me a patient had recently been admitted from the hospital with monitors still attached to their chest. She said,

> When we admitted the patient, we starting removing the monitors as the patient interrupted and said, "Wait! How are you going to monitor me without them?" The nurse paused, being struck by the question, and said, "we monitor you here with our eyes."

This example illustrates the struggle over understanding what being a hospice patient is like. For the patient, it made sense to have monitors attached to receive the proper care. Comparatively, the nurse practitioner struggled to define hospice experience as something other than having monitors attached to a person's body. In fact, monitoring patients with their eyes challenges other understandings of medical care at the end of life, which is often thought to include monitors, IVs, and other equipment.

A combined critical and dialogic perspective gives a distinct understanding of the dying experience. Even more, it reveals many ways that communication fosters particular meanings about death and dying, as the patient and nurse practitioner illustrated. This type of understanding moves beyond the "thick descriptions" (Geertz, 1973) that are characteristic of an interpretive approach, to actually asking researchers to take an ethical position with regard to the implications and messiness of communication, and their role in the mess. Therefore, distinguishing between interpretive and critical approaches will help you, the reader, better understand the goals of this study as well as some of my commitments. I borrow from Deetz (2001) a useful way of distinguishing between both approaches by describing the concepts of consensus and dissensus for understanding talk and its consequences in the ED and hospice.

According to Deetz (2001), scholars orienting near the consensus pole seek order and commonality. They treat order production as a dominant and natural feature of interaction. On the other hand, struggle, conflict, and tensions can be considered a natural state for understanding interaction (Zoller & Kline, 2008). Instead of focusing on describing and understanding realities, I am focusing on dissensus because I challenge dominant ways of knowing in the ED and hospice in order to uncover and reclaim hidden conflicts embedded in clinical talk. Therefore, my approach is rooted in voicing and acknowledging difference that helps bring a relational focus to a field often focused on message production. In short, my focus is towards the ongoing interaction where meaning is negotiated and produced within cultural contexts. As a result, I share an enduring interest in discourse, praxis, and language and the opportunities they hold for inspiring discussions around end of life, and helping to position us differently towards interactions with the ED and hospice.

Language is central to this study because it positions us to look at and respond to death in a particular way by forming relationships and distinctions, as well as making some things open to thought, examination, and discussion, and others not. This "positioning" is more than just having a set of beliefs or attitudes about health and illness though. Language, in fact, positions us to look at and respond to health and illness in a particular way (Deetz & Mumby, 1985). Therefore, a critical and dialogic perspective has given me tremendous sensitivity to how language is core to the process of constituting meaning around life and death, rather than simply naming what they are.

These sensitivities begin to bring awareness of how language and discursive formations control and prevent us from acting, thinking, and saying something different about life and death. Furthermore, they bring awareness of how the "particular ways of drawing on discursive formations as well as challenging and protecting them are all accomplished in actual interactions" (Deetz & Radford, 2008, p. 191). In other words, it brings awareness to the ways we struggle in interactions around end of life.

I have spent considerable time describing the ways in which meaning is produced. Next, I will describe what happens to meaning production when struggles persist and our talk becomes distorted. That is, when language closes the discussion or prevents discussions from taking place. Even more, shifting to the ways discourse becomes distorted is useful for understanding a subject like death, a subject we don't talk very much about. This next section will outline specific ways our talk leads to distortions, as well as ways our talk may begin opening important opportunities for communicating around end of life. Moving from the consequences of our talk to the opportunities it may hold is similar to thinking of the two options we have when we speak: we can talk to tell or we can talk to learn (Deetz & Radford, 2008).

Discursive Opening and Closing

To say that communication is the language of structural and system preferences is to also say that procedures, policies, practices, and even preferred ways of being become unable to be questioned or discussed (Deetz, 1992; Thackaberry, 2004). Therefore, I follow critical studies that argue distortion is an inevitable part of contemporary life.

According to Deetz (1992), a key to identifying and addressing discursive closure is examining interaction practices that privilege certain interests, meanings, and vocabularies over others. Specifically, I borrow from Deetz (1992) who outlines eight ways discourse becomes closed: neutralization, naturalization, subjectification of experience, pacification, topical avoidance, meaning denial, legitimation, and disqualification, many of which will be discussed later. These moves distort communication by suppressing "the unseen conflict in ways that appear to address the issues rather than suppress it" (Deetz & Radford, 2008, p. 191). More often than not, we use these strategies, and they use us, consciously and unconsciously. These forms of discourse act to distort power relations, disguise inequity, and oppress as well as emancipate us and our experiences (Clair, 1998). Said differently, communication can be silencing, especially around death and dying. To understand the dynamics of how communication becomes distorted and how communication silences, I borrow from Clair (1998) who asserts,

> Recognizing that discourse does more than communicate, realizing that discourses also articulate grand social systems, and discovering that discourses can silence certain people, specific issues, and particular interests, demands our attention. Of course,

we need to continue exploring how communication silences, but we also need to explore how silence communicates. (p. 39)

Therefore, the narratives we live by about life and death may speak of certain conditions while disguising others (Deetz, 1992). And some stories surrounding life and death may be expressed while others are sequestered (Clair, 1998). Further issues of power, culture, politics, aesthetics, and economics are all ways of explaining how language opens, closes, and distorts communication as well as how words and speech organize silence. The following example illustrates how communication becomes closed when established procedures at the end of life come into contact with a different culture whose access to language is distorted through a number of ways.

"Okay, let's go see this thing that I don't agree with," Doc says.

"Okay, but what's that?" I ask.

"The older woman who recently came in on the stretcher, the 95-year-old female from Russia."

My reflective experience: Getting closer to the room I see the 95-year-old with a mop of white hair, eyes shut, head tilted to the right and a breathing mask around her mouth, strapped behind her head, and a large clear tube connecting the mask to the machine helping her breathe. In a gray gown that was only visible above her chest and otherwise covered in a white hospital blanket. I thought "oh no" as we walked in.

"We have all the info we need," Doc tells the nurses. Holding the chart, Doc walks towards me and says,

"Look at it and tell me this doesn't seem absolutely ridiculous." The EMTs start gathering their things and say,

"Oh yeah, and she speaks 100% Russian. Absolutely no English but responds to pain and her name sometimes." Still trying to figure out what the chart says, Doc takes it back and says,

"95, do not resuscitate, needs a new G-tube to help her eat and drink. Can't speak English, pretty non-respondent. I would never make my family go through this." Doc looks at the EMTs and asks,

"When was the last time she has had fluids?"

"We think Friday," they say. And today is Monday. Shaking her head, Doc says,

"Friday! Food is one thing but with fluids she could die." I look at Doc and say,

"So she is DNR but without the tube she would die?"

"Well, she wouldn't be able to eat or drink so eventually yes," Doc says.

"And food through a G-tube means a sandwich or apple sauce?" I ask. Doc laughs and says,

"It depends but more like the latter." How is this DNR, I am thinking as we walk into the patient's room.

"Marlice! Marlice! How are you?" Doc says. No response as Doc walks closer and touches her arm. The patient turns her head slowly and opens her eyes but looks uncomfortable and exhausted. Doc keeps talking and rolls down the blanket and lifts her gown to expose the G-tube. Doc takes her stethoscope and begins moving it around her belly, pausing to listen. Marlice looks like she has fallen back to sleep. Still touching her belly with her bare hands, Doc looks up and says,

"It seems to be working just fine." I look at Doc and ask, "Can you ask her again if she wants this done?

"What do you mean?" Doc asks.

"Well, once something is decided can you ask them again?"

"Like being DNR?"

"Yeah. I mean this seems complicated if she is DNR when essentially she would die without this artificial tube."

"DNR is what I wish everyone would be! Unless of course someone like you who is young and healthy—we'd do everything we could. But DNR is the gold goal that I wish many would choose at this stage. So no, once the chart says it, I do what I am told and being Russian, she has strong cultural values about what to do."

"Crazy situation. So can you fix it or does someone have to come in?" I ask.

"Well I am going to put some fluids down to see if it is working properly first." I take several more looks at this 95-year-old who is essentially helpless, completely voiceless, without fluids or food for three days, who is here to have her tube fixed so she can drink and "eat" again. Doc is already at the computer as I stand outside the room for a minute longer pondering over this disturbing situation. I walk back to the computer where Doc is reading the patient's records and looks up and says,

"She has been in a lot and just five days ago they took a CT scan."

"Why?" I ask.

"Guess they wanted to check her belly."

"So without speaking English and a little unconscious, do you need to ask her for her consent?"

"Ask whether she wants one?"

"Yeah."

"No, we love scans here." I looked at Doc and slowly walked back to my post totally disturbed and confused. Doc walks over and says,

"I have an idea. Do you like coffee?"

"Yeah." She grabs her wallet and we walk to the café, passing the 95-year-old. I ordered a coffee and Doc ordered a raspberry scone. We walked back and I said,

"What would happen if you didn't fix the tube if you didn't believe that was 'right?'"

"That would never be an option. And I feel bad we are doing anything in the ER."

This interaction illustrates how distortions emerge at different moments of the interaction and can be cultural or systemic, like an institutional practice, or a suppression of a conflict closed off through language. Specifically, choice gets suppressed through both institutional regulations as well as cultural values in this interaction. Doc said, "once the chart says it, I do what I am told and being Russian, she has strong cultural values about what to do." Both the institutional practice of medical charting and the values embedded in Russian culture prevent a discussion from taking place and furthermore, close off any decision and course of action from critical engagement. The patient arrived unable to speak English and was pretty non-respondent. However, her previous chart listed DNR. Therefore, care practices and care decisions were already decided before the patient arrived, thereby influencing what the doctor could and could not do for her. Even more, these practices closed communication further since the patient could not verbally respond.

Communication, then, which is "open" refers to the ability of patients, families, and providers to question standardized procedures, meanings, practices, and even preferred ways of knowing around care.

This study will continue to illustrate how discourse, language, and silence organize meanings around end of life and how decisions with significant social, economic, political, physical, and emotional costs are coordinated around end of life. This focus takes language and struggle over meaning seriously. The complexities of how end of life is organized and in whose interests is it being organized, unfold through interaction.

Qualitatively describing the day-to-day emotional issues of patients, families, and providers and their interactions is necessary to make these issues come alive. Studies rich in detail, like this one, draw attention to language use. This attention makes a difference in how we understand talk in the ED and hospice. Further, we need to know how providers' work practices impact talk and how these same practices shape a particular orientation toward life and death. Finally, this study moves beyond simply understanding the dynamics and consequences of talk, to a sensitive critique of the way talk is organized at the ED and hospice. In doing so, this study will provide a deeper understanding of the way talk creates conversational openings and closures within these settings.

· 5 ·

THE COMPLEXITY OF DEATH
AT HOSPICE

In both the ED and hospice, death is chaotic. This is an enduring tension for life and work at both locations. Through organizational routines and practices, providers, patients, and families are able to tame temporarily, and therefore deal with, the complexity and messiness of death, as well as their own humanity.

Aspects of this tension are experienced from the first moment people arrive at either the ED or the hospice through an un-stripping of humanity that takes place. This un-stripping will become more clear as workers describe their experience of caring for patients in their last and most vulnerable moments of life. This un-stripping also comes from seeing patients at some of their most vulnerable moments, when everything we believed to matter in life is suddenly taken from us.

The tension is especially pressing at hospice, where staff see and experience this un-stripping while promoting, if not promising, that death is indeed different. This means living every moment to the fullest until you die. Seeing this un-stripping from any perspective can be horrifying, but is even more so when your role is to somehow promise that death is different in hospice. This chapter will focus on the hospice and the next one will focus on the ED.

In many ways, I experienced this tension when my idea of death slammed into my experience of death in the ED and the hospice. I did not know how to make it less chaotic or how to make sense of this tension, despite being familiar with many approaches to the way language works. But what I have discovered by listening, observing, and talking to providers is that they, too, experience this tension. And they manage it in fascinatingly different ways. Specifically, what follows are three ways that I believe providers handle this underlying tension between an un-stripping of humanity and the promotion of life and a good death at hospice. Embedded in each of these practices for managing this tension is a rehumanizing of their care practices.

Death is chaotic at hospice but daily routines help tame dying to allow what would otherwise be a disorderly place to remain perceptually orderly and coherent. Both professions—ED and hospice work—are helping and healing professions. We believe in these professions; we put great trust and faith in these professions and we turn to them when we are vulnerable, fragile, and need good care. These are sacred professions.

The first resolution surrounds the idea of rehumanizing death, which translates to transforming the actual work environment and work practices. The second resolution surrounds the notion of producing a difference, or a different quality of care at the end of life. And the final resolution becomes the active taming of death. Each resolution will be described in greater detail throughout the chapter. Importantly, these same resolutions will be used to illustrate how daily life is experienced in the ED. The resolutions may be similar, but the tension they are responding to is of a different flavor.

Transforming Work Practices

One way hospice manages the tension between an un-stripping of humanity and the promotion of a good death is by rehumanizing the dying process. Providers believe in this type of care so much that many of them believe they have been called to do this work. They have even taken significant pay cuts to work here. Even more, providers at hospice work to rehumanize death by transforming what it means to work at hospice and care for people who are dying. For example, when this hospice took over an old senior residence home, there was a sign on the nearby corner of 9th and Ellis Lane: "Dead End." Soon after the hospice began operation, the hospice petitioned to remove the sign. Though the hospice was unable to effect complete removal due to a city ordinance requiring information, the compromise was a sign that read: "Not a Through Street."

I start with this example because hospice is a place where workers assert they are different when attending to people who are dying. This was the first story I heard when beginning volunteer training at hospice. They start with this story because it asserts they are different and special at hospice, so much that the street sign needed to be changed. They don't want anyone to think that coming to hospice is a dead end. That language is too intense for a place designed to promote life and living, not death and dying. "Dead end" insists that turning on this street is synonymous with throwing in the towel and giving up. "Not a Through Street" leaves some space for hospice to promise that turning onto this street is not a death sentence but a place that takes you through death a little differently.

Even more, demanding this street sign be changed contributes to hospice workers defining who they are by how they are different, especially from a hospital setting. This different way of attending to the dying includes their focus on listening, embracing life, and managing symptoms to keep patients comfortable. The difference they seek is produced through the language they use and the stories they tell, specifically when describing their motivation for working at hospice.

Rehumanizing death deals with transforming the actual meaning of their work and their role in the dying process. For example, Larry, the chaplain, says,

A good day is when in that process, during visiting, something opens up with family members or with a patient that takes us to a deeper level, a deep level of encounter, or of conversation about something that really truly is needed in their spiritual life. I look for completion, and for closure on some things.

This passage is interesting in the way it transforms an interaction with a patient into an encounter that takes the patient and provider to a place they need to be. Transforming the interaction into a deep-level encounter turns it further into a task where completion becomes something to be achieved. Also interesting is how this encounter attempts to rehumanize death by pointing out that there is something lost and therefore needed for this patient in their spiritual life. And this something becomes a way for this particular provider to regain closure and transform what it means to interact with a patient who is dying by seeking closure, which seems to be doing more for the provider in their attempt to rehumanize death.

Another example of how providers resolve their underlying tension is ev-
ident as they attempt to manage the emotional state around death by trying
to change the way individuals think about death. For example, Larry goes on
to say,

> We are not trying to fix something; we're trying to fix somebody's way of looking at
> things. And the ability to do that comes from some place that I am not always sure
> where that is. But something within me is awareness, knowledge, and experience that
> I draw on that everything will be OK. All will be well. Whatever the outcome is in
> our minds, all will be well.

The attempt to fix somebody's way of looking at things is central at hospice.
The acceptance, however, of seeing death as something else takes tremendous
work by the provider, patient, and family. And it even takes a leap of faith
that all will be well no matter what is happening. Believing that all will be
right relieves tremendous pressure from describing how potentially difficult
and threatening it is to be at hospice. It is as if nothing else can matter so long
as we engage others with the idea that everything will be all right. This, too,
helps rehumanize death into something not too scary but something that can
be managed through a belief that all will be well. Rehumanizing death is also
described as part of their jobs as providers; one nurse shared:

> One of the things we do here is we spend a lot of time talking to people. It is one of
> our fortes, so to speak. And it often takes several meetings with them to emphasize
> and reinforce certain principles or whatever it is that we're trying to reinforce. To re-
> ally try to hear them out and to get to know them, and I think in our current structure
> of how we receive health care that that's not always possible. So I think a lot of what
> I hear when people get to hospice is that they haven't had things explained to them
> in that way, or they wish they could have come to hospice sooner.

The focus on listening is interesting for a few reasons and is used again to help
produce the belief that a hospice experience is different from another hospital
experience. Listening, however, seems to take a particular path in that even
while it becomes a forte of theirs, it is clear that they listen for specific things
or listen in order to achieve certain things. The nurse above talks about how
it can take several meetings to "reinforce certain principles" but those certain
principles are less clear. Listening, too, becomes a way for hospice workers to
distinguish themselves as different from other forms of care that are familiar
to patients and families. And her last sentence underscores that the rest of
the healthcare system is lacking something that hospice has. Some of the

principles I believe they are trying to reinforce are connected to rehumanizing death. For example, another nurse describes her way of transforming death into something else when she says,

> Part of my job is to help normalize the dying process and make it not so scary for people. It can be a really beautiful time in somebody's life too; it can be a lot of sharing and really connecting with patients. But most of us white folk just don't acknowledge it and don't embrace it like they often do in different cultures.

Believing that death is something other than horrific, painful, and devastating helps people cope, especially at hospice. But the idea of transforming death into something beautiful is not easily accepted. In fact, it becomes difficult for providers too, as one nurse shared,

> Caring for anybody in a hospital, hospice, or nursing home setting is tiring because we are people. We don't work on clockwork like computers. You can't take a break when you want to. You don't always get a lunch break because my role is to take care of patients and have their symptoms managed. I can't go to lunch if I have someone in severe pain. That is not who I am and why I am here.

This passage really underscores the tensions of transforming the environment at hospice in an attempt to rehumanize death. At the start, the nurse describes how exhausting working in any medical setting is and reminds us all that they are people too who must manage the demands of this kind of setting. She goes on to describe some of the things that make it tiring but she does so in relationship to her role at hospice: to manage symptoms. It's as if she begins to feel guilty for describing how demanding and exhausting it is because that is not who she is or why she is there. The transforming of the work environment and her role in it works to suppress some of the noticeable challenges of doing this work.

Another example of the struggle to rehumanize death involves the role of emotions and their role in the dying process. In the following example, the chaplain describes how this work is challenging yet describes it as something more meaningful than challenging. He says,

> I do grieve. Some patients that we lose, the ones that die, I do grieve because I like to be close and have some chemistry with them. And I have become profoundly aware of grief in people's lives and resonate with that sometimes. So I cry a lot. And that's okay. The tears are part of the journey and they are important because they are expressive of the profound and expressive of the loss we all feel in this life. Life is tough and it's hurtful and there is a lot of pain in the journey. And I don't see any

reason to keep from experiencing it. So I think it is important to let myself have the tears occasionally.

Part of rehumanizing death walks a fine line between believing death to be something else, yet needing to explain the reason for specific feelings, like tears. For the chaplain, tears here become understood as an expressive act of the difficulties of life. But it is as if there is guilt in feeling otherwise, as the last sentence describes how he lets himself have the tears occasionally. Work is tough at hospice. It is demanding emotionally, spiritually, and physically. But attempting to rehumanize death requires a rethinking of the job and role at hospice. One way that seems to help providers cope with rehumanizing death is transforming the meaning of their job. For example, one nurse shared:

> If you love your job and you're not getting raises or benefits, it's not tempting to stay. But for some people like me, it is because I wouldn't want to be at a mediocre job where I didn't feel passionate about my work. Or if it was a job that was OK and every day was the same. It's repetitive even though I would be getting more money with better benefits, it doesn't give the same self-satisfaction as working here.

This is not an uncommon remark for providers at hospice: working here gives providers satisfaction. And being close to people dying brings satisfaction. But in order to rehumanize death, it makes sense that the work environment and their work practices must also be transformed and therefore rehumanized. Believing that death is beautiful and not scary requires a set of practices. Specifically, if those things are to be achieved at hospice, providers must believe in those things and one way to do that is by believing in their work and believing that their work is satisfying and meaningful. And during the moments where providers talk about the challenges and demands of this work, it often gets reframed as part of the process or an expression of life at hospice.

Rehumanizing death allows providers and patients to contemplate their role. It also helps transform meanings surrounding what it is like to care for people who are dying. These meanings around listening, feeling satisfied, believing they are part of deep encounters, become ways for hospice workers to continue producing this difference, so that they are indeed different from any hospital experience. Other ways that hospice attempts to rehumanize death are through actual activities such as the hospitality cart or "cocktail cart"; live music and entertainment; music therapy; massage and aromatherapy treatments; pet therapy with visiting dogs and llamas; and art classes. Each of these, in turn, helps to rehumanize death in ways that honestly distract patients and families from their impending condition. They also work to organize a different meaning of quality during the end of life. The struggles to produce this difference surround the second tension of producing a different meaning of quality of days at the end of life.

A Different Ethics of Care

A second way that providers manage the tension of promoting a good death in a place that endlessly strips away part of humanity is through the belief that hospice is unique and different. Even more, hospice talk shapes meaning that somehow this place is different from another medical experience. Although the difference is never explicitly stated, part of the difference surrounds how hospice organizes a particular meaning of quality at the end of life. Part of organizing a new meaning of quality involves describing how quality of days at the end of life is a unique experience. One nurse describes this by saying:

> Being able to really change somebody's end of life care from being in the hospital with tubes that they really didn't want, to be comfortable here, bring them a cocktail at 4pm or whatever makes them happy. Just to be able to give them the quality instead of just more days. Being able to control symptoms seems more rewarding. It's patients and what you do for the patients. It's hugely rewarding. I think the whole IDT (interdisciplinary team) approach is huge. Maybe medically we can't address it, but maybe the chaplains can with spirituality, or maybe we can with music or aromatherapy or being able to use all these tools to help people transition peacefully.

This passage helps illustrate how this particular provider's talk works to describe some of the very things they believe in and do in order to organize a new meaning of quality. In fact, at times it seems like their particular understanding of quality becomes something to believe in, accept, and act upon in order to think about death differently.

Understanding quality becomes about understanding it as different from being in the hospital with tubes. Because quality at hospice is less about time or quantity and more about what hospice thinks is more meaningful: choice in having things that are often lost in a hospital setting. Another way quality is produced and organized here is through their focus on a team-based approach that allows them to deliver care that is different and unique. Producing a different kind of quality that allows patients to transition peacefully during the last days is illustrated further when another nurse shares that,

> Hospice is kind of a whole different focus because most nursing you're trying to fix a problem or make their disease better or get rid of the infection, fix their broken bones or something restorative. Whereas hospice, you have to do a whole different mind shift. It's not fixing. You're going to let the natural disease progress, and you're going to manage their symptoms and help them live every day that they have here. This is instead of just being miserable, depressed, and sick and in pain. It's a totally different mind shift in nursing but I think it is very challenging and very rewarding.

Not fixing the problem is an important distinction and important struggle at hospice for providers and patients. Nurses and patients are used to "fixing" or being "fixed" and both seem to struggle accepting something other. A better word at hospice might be to "tame," which means letting the natural disease progress as it may. Quality here is again described as being able to help patients and families live every day that they have here, rather than live more days. Further yet, quality is described and understood as something different from another hospital setting experience, which is understood to be miserable, depressing, sick, and painful.

The way providers resolve this tension is further illustrated in the quickness to first describe the challenges of this work, followed shortly thereafter by the rewards and gratifications of the work at hospice. Embracing quality becomes important because it allows providers to believe that their work is not only different but also meaningful enough to sustain them through the difficult task of caring for the dying. Hospice clearly affects people; if nothing else it gives those who come close an entirely new perspective not only about death, but also about life.

Part of this new perspective is a result of being at hospice every day and listening, hearing, feeling, and seeing things that happen at the end of life. For example, one nurse explained that there had been six or seven weddings in the last six months at hospice. She said,

> I mean, driving out of the parking lot and seeing a young woman—also a patient—walking down the aisle…I mean you just don't see that anywhere. The point is now they are married and that's what they wanted and it's fantastic. It'd be better to say I did it than what would it have been like if I didn't do it? I would rather live with fewer regrets than take a chance. You just see other people happy when you see them make the choice to finally live. Because it is not about dying, it's not about death. It's living your life to the very end and living it how you want to.

Again, quality here becomes understood as enjoying what time patients have left rather than trying to lengthen the stay. And in this case, a patient deciding to get married while in hospice is a way providers see and feel the difference of this experience, especially around quality of days at the end of life.

Even more, this particular nurse quickly makes sense of a patient deciding to get married because that's what it is about here, taking a chance to live. And in some ways, deciding to get married and hospice supporting that helps to maintain the belief and practice that this is not about death and dying. Rather, it is about living and having some choice at the end of life to do things that matter to the patient and to the provider. For this nurse to see a wedding while driving home from work does something to her. After watching it, she said she would rather live with fewer regrets. Organizing a particular understanding of quality of days during the end of life seems to also translate to understanding quality of days during providers' own lives. Working at hospice to produce a different kind of quality at the end of life makes providers aware and reflexive of other things when interacting with patients. For example, one nurse said,

> You are going to want to really step up and be a person of your word. If I say I am going to be back in five minutes, you better be back in five minutes, not 10 or 30. People really value your word especially here. They don't have a lot of time to argue with you. They don't have a lot of time in this world to have false promises. You have to be really conscientious of how you make promises.

I felt a similar pressure to really step up as a volunteer. The idea of quality of life and letting someone die more peacefully than at another place, puts certain demands on people who work there to do something different, or even something better.

I, too, was conscious of my word, thinking what if this patient isn't here next time I come back? Or what if my bringing them Cheetos or a glass of chocolate milk is the last thing they will taste before they die? Do they really need ice in their juice? But what if this is the last orange juice they will sip? Is it necessary I drive to the Safeway to buy organic lemons for a patient who wants to make a picnic in her room and sip lemonade with natural citrus? Did my decision change knowing her time is limited? These become enormous expectations, and it makes sense why quality over quantity matters so much. You have to be a person of your word and patients don't have a lot of time in this world to have false promises. As a result, these become big commitments to maintain within an environment that pushes and pulls people in different directions about the meaning of life and death. Even though this felt like enormous work and responsibility for me, providers were quick to remind me and others that this is what hospice is all about. Specifically, Gerry told me,

> All you have to do to work with people at the end of life is listen. I mean there's other things that you do, but that's the most important thing, just to listen to people. Just to be with people and not to abandon them and say that you can't help them because you can help them. So essentially it's very simple. It's very easy to take care of people at the end of life. You just have to listen to them.

> Listening seems rather straightforward, but for anyone who does listen well, especially to people who are very sick and are believed to be dying, listening empathetically is not always easy.

It certainly was challenging for me to hear the tremble of voices, the mumbles, mutters, silences, stories, tangents, and the soft and shaky comments that they wished they were someplace else. Those voices and stories are hard to listen to. But it makes a difference at hospice, just like their purpose to "not abandon" patients. Whenever a patient is put "on watch" there is always someone, like a volunteer, in the room to just "be" with the patient while they die. Listening and just being are not characteristic of a hospital setting. Therefore, these practices become ways to further illustrate how quality is understood differently at hospice. It is a rethinking of what being a provider at hospice means—or even an undoing, according to one nurse who said,

> Coming to hospice, you are undoing everything you did in nursing. It's not treat the diabetes, treat the high cholesterol with diet and exercise. It's eating what you want, you don't have to take your insulin, or your medications. So you go from one extreme to the next. With pain medication in the hospital, you can have pain medication every four hours, like Percocet and Vicodin. Here it is every one hour. So nurses in the field who aren't educated in hospice are a little skeptical about giving morphine and high dosage narcotics every hour because they are in that old morphine fears that if they give this dose they are doing to die. Restrictive environments like hospitals and ERs are not very liberal with the pain medication and anxiety medicine like we are.

Part of the undoing of what nurses and providers have learned elsewhere seems less about moving from one extreme to another than it is about producing a different understanding of quality of days at the end of life.

At hospice, a number of things are used to bring comfort to patients and families, including pain medication. There are many ways of understanding how hospice is different, from providers telling you that it is a whole different way of providing care, to being something very easy, if you just listen. The focus on producing a new understanding of quality of days, however, remains the same. Producing this difference no doubt influences those who work, volunteer, visit, or care for people at hospice.

Organizing a particular meaning of quality surrounding days at the end of life creates a tension, however, because many patients are endlessly confused and uncertain about what hospice is, but often feel that it is something different from what they've experienced, even peaceful and special. This favorable view gets communicated to the public, who begin thinking too that hospice is a special and wonderful place. This is not bad, obviously, but it positions people to see certain things at the expense of others, often the less beautiful things taking place. But this unique talk in many ways serves as a coping and numbing device for the sadness and confusion surrounding death. More, believing in the uniqueness of the place seems to open the possibility that death is something other than terrible and sad. In short, it helps to tame the wildness surrounding death at hospice.

Taming Death

The final way providers manage this underlying tension is through the language they use to tame death or bring death into control. Specifically, the language of religion and spirituality works to tame the wildness surrounding death for patients, families, and providers. As will be clear in the examples below, this type of language provides a comforting frame of reference for many while at the same time providing a rather narrow vocabulary and set of explanations for what is happening. Essentially, this tension becomes a sense-making device for patients, providers, and families. Our language is believed to be limited surrounding death so it is no wonder hospice providers and patients turn to spirituality and religion to make sense of the situation. The point, however, is to understand what using this type of language does for providers and patients, rather than to believe how it should look or sound different.

One nurse, for example, describes how death can look different from what people imagine because she sees God working every day here. She shared,

> Growing up I went through a lot of spiritual paths, being raised Presbyterian then having my mom die, having multiple other people die, I really became agnostic, and not very connected with God or source, or spiritual whatever you say. And through nursing, actually hospice really brought me back to my source, spirit, God. Huge belief because I see it all the time. I see God working with lives, see them talking to angels, or fixed on the light. It's part of the circle of life, and that's one thing you're

not going to get out of: nothing that is living ever dies so why be scared of that? If you do have a strong connection with God or some spirituality, I think death is not a scary thing but kind of just challenging.

Believing and seeing God work at hospice help her cope with the difficulties of death and try to bring some control to an uncertain experience. At the end of this passage, she underscores that if people have a strong connection with God or some spirituality, death is not a scary thing. She does admit it is challenging, but believing in something greater than the self helps her cope with death and dying. It is much easier to imagine seeing God working than the devil, even though it felt like that sometimes for me. Our meanings surrounding spirituality and religion provide a more peaceful and comforting reference for death. It helps gives us an explanation to make sense of what is taking place. Just as it has been said before, even working to view death as something other than scary is not to say that it makes the work any easier. One nurse told me,

> You have to really go home and feel good about what you are doing. And I think 99% of the staff does. But it can take a toll on your personal well-being at home. You go home feeling very sad and depressed about things.

I was no exception to feeling this way as a consequence of being there and my time was significantly limited compared to the providers doing this work. The tension between taming death and experiencing death is further illustrated and felt; another nurse told me,

> You deal with death and dying and the potential of death and dying every day. So how do you get up every morning and think about your patients who have done everything right and they are still sick. Or the patients who haven't done anything right and they are sick. How do you go home and figure I should eat right, I should exercise when I have two patients that did everything right and they still have terminal diagnosis? How do you do that? I think you go home and you love your children more, you appreciate things more. But it can certainly be mentally unhealthy. That's why we have our bereavement groups that are offered to the staff so we can talk about patients and things that maybe we had a difficult time with.

There seems to be a disconnect between what people say death and dying are at hospice and what people experience as a consequence of being and working at hospice. Part of the taming, then, seems to become untamed in other ways, like people's personal life where you start loving more deeply, and question what you eat and how you exercise.

Some of the other ways language works to tame death are heard and felt during my interview with Larry when he said,

> Death is not a mystery to solve but a mystery to be involved in. And it's just something that in general, as family members experience the dying process, occasionally I'll get a chance to hear them say, 'I just don't know why she has to suffer so much. What did she do, or he do that he's suffering so much? Or maybe he brought this on himself anyway. After all he was a drunk, he was a drug user, maybe he is getting what he deserves but it doesn't seem fair to me!' And you know those are good comments that someone has to wrestle through with. But it also has this kind of cause and effect orientation that God is devising this onto the person or they're reaping what they sowed.

This is interesting because at the very moment people are really struggling and wrestling with important questions, these struggles become understood through a cause and effect orientation to bring some control to a set of questions that seem out of control to have to process. Larry went on to say,

> What is going on in the dying process is so much greater than that and so much is mysterious. And it's something to wonder at. It's going to be painful, it's not that it is not painful to watch or painful to experience. Although with our medications we cut down on the pain aspect of it.

This passage helps illustrate a contradiction at hospice about believing death to be something natural, peaceful, and beautiful, as providers struggle to handle the chaos and uncertainty of the process. They are quick to share that death is indeed painful to watch and experience, but their talk seems to promote another understanding that helps bring control to these other feelings surrounding death. Another way that death is tamed at hospice is illustrated when a nurse shares a recent interaction she had with a patient's family about death and the status of the patient. She mentioned before how important it is to convey information calmly and compassionately about the normal progress of the disease and dying process, when sometimes it's very difficult when providers know it's not that way. Specifically, she said,

> You tell them they are getting pain medication and you have to be honest: your mom, your dad, or your brother is getting more pain medicine. We've talked to the doctor and increased their dosage. Sure they are physically changing we can see that, which means we are moving along in the disease process. And you have to be the one who kind of says it or they'll say I know what the answer is going to be can you please just tell me? Are they imminently dying? Are they dying the next day? And you know they are.

After she stopped here, I asked if she does tell the family the truth. She answered,

> You do. You know you say, they are on watch and they are imminently dying. They don't have a lot of time left. But what I can do for you now while you are here to help you get through the process? Like what can I do? I will manage your loved one based on their symptoms to make sure they are calm, peaceful, and comfortable. What can I do for you? Have you had enough to eat today? Have you rested? Make sure you go walk. Can I bring you something to drink? Can I call someone for you? Because once they know it is the end, the end without a doubt, people tend to become very shut down and quiet or very almost relieved.

The passage is interesting in how it moves quickly after saying the patient is imminently dying to focusing on the family or those in the room. Questions about what hospice can do for them are interesting in that they seem to remove the focus for a minute from the patient who is dying to making sure now the family is comfortable.

These honest gestures work to bring calm during a time that is often filled with agitation. Questions about dying are answered here by way of how providers can bring comfort to family as well. Another interesting experience of how providers tame death surrounds what it means to work here. For example, one nurse described working at hospice through a fascinating comparison. She said,

> It's the most rewarding job I've ever had. I put it in the fact of the circle of life. When babies are born, they come into this world at the place, time, and family they want to. You're born to this world when you want to be. And you leave this world when you want to with the people who you want around you or not around you. And it's the same philosophy. Family is at the bedside when their baby is born, it's joyous, it's happy. Family is at the beside when someone is dying too. It's not joyous and happy but your family is still there from the beginning until the end. So is it less fulfilling when a person takes their last breath or the last person they see or hear or feel or touch? Is it less rewarding than bringing someone into this world as a nurse in OB? It's the same kind of thing…Nobody ever says to an OB nurse, isn't your job sad and depressing or awful or terrible? How do you bring someone into this world with all the problems? That's supposed to be in our culture a joyous, happy time but the dying process is supposed to be a bereaving, sad, grief-stricken, depressing time. So we need to change the education to the nursing staff, health care professionals, and families that this is not a time of sadness and horrific tragedy.

Comparing death to birth is useful to again bring some control and explanation to the dying process. Understanding death within the circle of life, however, puts much control on the person to be able to choose when they want to come into this world and therefore leave this world. It doesn't seem so straightforward.

Would some babies really choose to be born with a degenerative disability or to a parent on drugs? Similarly, would some people really choose to die at age 25 or choose to leave the world not knowing who the people around their bed are? At hospice, it seems useful to understand life and death within broader cultural understandings, like the circle of life. In doing so, it helps to tame what otherwise would be out of control to understand. At hospice, language shapes meanings surrounding death as something other than wild or chaotic. By transforming care practices to actively seek to produce a different meaning of quality surrounding the last days of life, language here tames death.

Taming, however, does not remove the wildness of it; rather, it displaces the wildness of death so as to not have to manage it directly. In other words, the wildness of death is suppressed through talk, work practices, and even material artifacts similar to the example about the sign, "Not a Through Street" that opened this chapter. Suppressing and displacing death at hospice enables providers, patients, and families to achieve certain goals. At the same time, however, displacing the wildness surrounding death also constrains them from achieving and understanding other things as well. This matters because through organizational routines and practices, providers, patients, and families are able to tame and therefore deal with the messiness of death as well as their own humanity. But what gets lost or constrained when the complexity around death gets suppressed?

The ways of managing the underlying tension at hospice are broad but intersect in interesting and important ways. Death is certain. Moreover, it doesn't make good sense and is hard to understand. But both hospice and the ED staff work to make sense of it. Listening to providers gives a glimpse into their worlds, every day in the face of life and death. Notable, however, are the meanings they struggle with at work and the ways they bring order to an otherwise disorderly place.

Work in both places is difficult, exhausting, and demanding. In both places, though, work becomes organized to bring some control, albeit through different means, to the dying process. Essentially at hospice, providers' talk attempts to rehumanize death and, therefore, their work environment. This transforming of care practices further produces a difference in quality of care and quality of days at the end of life. This difference becomes important because through behaviors, the language of spirituality and religion, seeing someone choose to get married, listening, the belief that caring for people who are dying is easy, and the satisfaction of being with people at the end of life, death becomes tamed. But it is clear that working to tame death at hospice lets it out in other places, like providers' personal lives. It raises the question, what happens to our understanding of death and life when we work to bring them both under control?

Working at hospice, seeing and hearing the things behind the main doors, moves people in certain ways. Do you gain a new perspective on death? Do you gain a new perspective on life? Does working at hospice affect providers' own personal relationships? Does it make you rethink your actions and decisions based on what you experienced as a consequence of being at hospice? Do you remain the same after being here?

The next chapter will describe how ED providers achieve order in a chaotic environment through discourse.

· 6 ·

THE MESSINESS OF DEATH IN THE EMERGENCY DEPARTMENT

The rhythm in the ED is fast, loud, busy, and chaotic. Waiting rooms can be crowded and time can be pressing, yet providers struggle to make a difference in their care. And therein lies the tension. EDs follow a set of organizational practices and protocols. But at the same time a multitude of patients, conditions, and symptoms are to be cared for within tight time constraints. Therefore, providers struggle to manage the tension between following rigid time protocols and the sheer volume of patients, while providing care that responds to the unique circumstances of an individual's life and health. In short, they struggle to make a difference in a system that endlessly suppresses differences through protocols, checklists, and standards. In their struggle, they manage this tension creatively by transforming their care practices.

In order to let you see and feel how life is at the ED, I have organized ED workers' experiences around three ways of managing this tension, parallel to that at hospice. First, the providers manage the tension by their own ways of rehumanizing care practices that ultimately transform the work environment towards a specific purpose. Second, the providers refashion a different meaning of quality care that becomes more about time and trying to save patients rather than simply keeping them comfortable. Finally, they manage the tension by transforming care practices and refashioning quality, in light of the purpose in the ED that ultimately works to tame death.

These resolutions, like those at hospice, work to bring order to a disorderly environment and experience. More, the ways providers manage this tension between individualized care and strict time and patient volume work to control death. Each of the ways providers manage this tension will be described in greater detail throughout this chapter, based on providers' experiences and stories. I will begin with the third form of resolution, transforming work practices, by starting with a story of delivering bad news in the ED. I am choosing to start here in part because it highlights the tension I am talking about in the ED between delivering care within rigid standards and protocols and being able to attend to the unique circumstances of an individual's life and health.

Transforming Work Practices

The ED is organized with a specific purpose in mind: bring patients in, fix them, and send them on their way. Although this purpose is useful, the ED must be flexible enough to deal with a multitude of patients and conditions. Therefore, the multiple conditions and circumstances run in opposition to simply fixing and sending patients on their way, especially within strict time constraints. To begin to feel this struggle, take the following story that an ED doctor sent to me verbatim over email:

The 54-year old woman looked tired but she had just gotten off a plane from Europe with her husband. They were sent in by their doctor for evaluation of sharp chest pain and shortness of breath. He was concerned about a possible blood clot in her lung after the long plane trip. I embarked on the usual workup for this including the CT scan of her chest. The busy shift made it impossible to stay on top of all the patients. The red phone from the radiologist rang. The reading on the CT was back.

"Yes," I said. "That patient is mine." I listened to the reading. My face did not reveal what I just heard. A nurse asked me to discharge a patient who was getting frustrated with their length of stay; an ambulance arrived with another patient. I listened to their report with minimal attention. I was thinking about what I needed to do next.

As I approached Room 6, I could see the middle-aged couple laughing about something he was reading in the paper by her bedside. My pace slowed as I knew that what I was about to say would change their life. My shoulders slumped a little but I took a deep breath and sat at her bedside.

I reached out and placed my hand on her leg. Was it to ground her or me, I wondered? "I have the results of the CT scan. This will be difficult to hear." I intellectually knew that there was a way in which to prepare the patient but I felt like I forgot it all in that moment.

"While you do have a blood clot in your lungs, it is rather small and can be treated with medicine that will prevent more clots from forming as your body breaks this one down. But what is more concerning is that your breast cancer that you had appears to have returned and has spread to your chest, liver and bones." I stop talking. I continue to touch her leg and I watch her husband move to her shoulder. Her eyes turn from me and well up. Her lip quivers and then the corners turn down ever so slightly. I feel myself let out a breath, not even realizing I had been holding it, forgetting to exhale.

In that moment, the joy of their trip and the rest of their lives that they had planned vaporized. I heard my name paged for the third time. I continued to ignore it. And I just sat with them. "I am going to step out and give you some time and then I will return and we can talk some more about what this means. I am going to have the nurse get your medicine started for the blood clot. I am sorry to give you this news." I step out of the room. I want to turn the other way and walk right out the back doors of the ER. But I round the corner of the nurse's station and sign orders on a couple of charts and walk into Room 14 to suture a laceration from a glass of wine that broke. "Emergent ambulance Room 1." I glance up relieved to see one of the other docs walk in behind the paramedics. I go back to suturing the wound. I wish that all wounds could be managed so easily.

I choose this example because it illustrates the tension in the ED around providing care in this type of environment. Furthermore, it brings attention to the way providers struggle to care for patients in an environment that demands so much from them, yet doesn't always support their needs. Even more, it illustrates how the ED is organized to keep providers doing many different things at once, often under strict time constraints. But this example also underscores the struggle for providers to attempt to rehumanize care practices in the ED. In the example, you can feel the tension, struggle and frustration of having to give this news as she is being paged, for the third time, to go see another patient with a laceration from a glass of wine. This pattern happens frequently in the ED.

Part of the tension surrounds the belief that not many people can really understand what goes on in the ED without being there. I think not being able to understand is an attempt to appreciate some of the difficulties providers experience working in a place like this and struggling against their own humanity. For example, the same physician describes working here as follows:

> The ED is really quite unique and unless you get to really witness it and witness the personalities and know the people, and know that they are not jerks and not callous, then you start to see it from a different perspective that is all part of how we manage and continue to show up every day and carry the burden with us of pain, suffering, and acute problems.

The passage again works to help rehumanize ED practices. Even the point that providers are not callous jerks sets up this tension around what they are expected to do in the ED and what they experience in the ED. Part of rehumanizing care practices to disprove that the providers are jerks often comes out by describing what happens in the ED and what they are called to do. Knowing and hearing some of these stories will help us all rethink what it means and what it feels like working here. For example, one nurse shared this story:

> The last time I worked we had a 35-year-old girl that had history of brain cancer. She was three years out, she thought she was clear. She came in vomiting and she's like, 'I'm afraid there's a brain tumor.' And I'm like, 'well, maybe it's just a virus. Why don't we wait and see.' She had seven brain tumors. And we had to go in and tell this girl you have terminal brain cancer.

Delivering this kind of news is not uncommon in the ED, but points to the tension surrounding its environment. Specifically, it is as if providers feel like the ED is a "funny" place to have to give this kind of news. That somehow, it shouldn't have to happen this way, within an environment that is constantly shifting between patients' needs that are truly critical to providers and those that only seem critical to patients. For example, when a patient came in with a sore throat after another patient had just died. The physician said,

> But you know that's not their problem. Their life is what matters to them and their illness affecting them. Sometimes you have to say something when they're really rude to you about how long they have had to wait and I have to say you know what, I needed to tend to somebody who is critical and I would hope that you or when your own family member are in that position, you would want us to make that a priority as well. I am sorry that it doesn't feel like we are attending to your need but in the emergency room it is truly based on critical need first. But you know, the short translation of that is, 'fuck you,' you know. Who do you think you are is how it comes out with anger when you're tired. It's like where do you get off thinking you are so important, but you can't say that. Well, sometimes I do but I get in trouble.

This again illustrates the challenges of rehumanizing care in the ED for those patients considered "emergent" all the while still attending to those who believe their condition is "emergent." The ED is a place where any and all conditions must be treated. Therefore, it puts relentless pressure on providers to make a difference in an environment that is endlessly changing.

Despite the difference, providers attempt to rehumanize the challenges of working in the ED as well as the frustrations. For example, a caseworker shared how conversations can be difficult with patients, especially patients with drug or alcohol addictions. She said,

> You feel like you're not getting anywhere. You're just talking to yourself, you're having that same conversation, and it's frustrating. I've had patients that I just see repeatedly and it's frustrating. They are back in here constantly because they're not doing what they're supposed to be doing. And I don't know how to help them.

The frustration in her voice describes the difficulty of making a difference for patients who frequent the ED. Even more, it is understood within an environment where providers do feel overworked, frustrated, and tired. One of the challenges of rehumanizing care in the ED is the steady workflow; one nurse describes a bad day as follows:

> A bad day is when we're crazy busy and we don't have enough staff. And we're just running our butts off and I get home and my day is still playing in my head because it was a horrible busy day.

In some ways, this passage relates back to the first example of delivering bad news within an environment that produces a rhythm that requires stamina and constant shifting of focus and emotion. Even more, it requires providers to be somewhat autonomous in providing care as one nurse shared:

> If you start falling behind and you have a medication at 07:00 and you don't document it until 11:30 legally speaking if anything were to happen to that patient court records could come back and say you didn't, it says you said 07:00 but the chart says 11:30. What time was it really done? And there's ways to overcome that through our charting process but it's best to stay on top of it. But to remember everything that you've done and to be working with these patients, one person's ringing the bell and this person needs to go for a scan.

Feeling satisfied, then, is difficult in a system as regulated as the ED, where providers are tired after working a twelve-hour shift. Feeling overworked and underappreciated constrains providers from becoming emotionally invested in every patient. In fact, sometimes it is difficult as one nurse describes after meeting a patient during her shift:

> The first thing he said to me when I walked in the door was, 'give me a fuckin' sandwich.' That was the first thing he said to me. Not hello, not hey, and I said whoa! I was like, 'my name is Kelly, and I'm your nurse.' And he's like, 'I pay your salary, get me a fuckin' sandwich.' And I said, 'no you don't. I have not worked for the government for a very long time, and by the looks of you, you have not paid taxes for a very long time. So you don't pay my salary, sir. And the last thing you're going to get from me talking to me like that is a sandwich. Now, would you like to rephrase that?' And he's like, 'may I please have a sandwich?' 'Absolutely you can have a sandwich, yes.' And from then on it was okay, but it was really hard for me to really care about that man, and care about whether or not he got home, you know. I got him a sandwich and that was like the end of my emotional investment in that person.

This passage underscores the difficulty of providing care in the ED, specifically how invested providers can become. Although it seems as though rehumanizing care practices within the ED is something to strive for, these practices often stay at a standstill because of the way the environment is organized towards a specific purpose.

Essentially, the ED is often considered a place to go in emergent situations where the goal for providers is to do less talking and more saving lives. Even more, the purpose is organized around bringing patients stability and relief until providers decide where the patient needs to go to get further care. In this sense, EDs can be seen as "transition" or "saving" places where patients who need critical care can come for immediate help. Interestingly, however, EDs are becoming more of "dumping places" for anyone who needs mental, physical, emotional, and spiritual care, thereby putting great pressure on the meaning of emergency and the organization of emergency medicine's purpose.

This leads to the second way providers attempt to manage the tension of transforming the meaning of quality care. The above examples help you feel what it is like to experience the ED from a provider's perspective: It's challenging and exhausting. Even more, a struggle emerges between wanting to provide care that is more customized, unique, and humanized, but having to do so within a system organized to achieve efficient, effective, and sophisticated care. The latter characteristics put pressure on the meaning of quality of care in the ED, as well as the meaning of quality of life for providers' own experience.

A Different Quality of Care

Much of the ED is organized around protocols and standards of care. It is also organized so that providers must constantly be moving and multi-tasking. At any given moment, much like some of the earlier examples given, providers are hearing pages over the intercom, observing and listening to the monitors, watching patient rooms, transferring patients, ordering labs, receiving lab results, making phone calls, communicating with other colleagues, and charting, among other things. These tasks are not always well compensated, and they make a difference in the attitude and willingness of providers to become involved in what is going on that day in the ED.

To deal with some of the complexities surrounding the multitude of tasks that providers perform, they use certain devices, like sarcasm, or emphasize the importance of working with good people, to manage the complexities in the ED. Time becomes both a barrier to patient care and a way to structure providers' own thoughts and feelings. For example, when describing what makes a good day a physician shared,

> A good shift is if we can have food and we can play practical jokes on each other and for me, we have a lot of fractures that I can fix like where you can have a simple thing where they come in, you can identify the issues and fix it. That is satisfying. It's not super satisfying to manage chronic diseases because it feels like you're not really affecting anything—you're just sort of throwing a little water on some flames and damping it down. It does feel good when you have someone that sprains their ankle, breaks their wrist and you can fix it, or sew it up. Even if they have a heart attack and you take them to the CATH lab, you identified something and you can fix it. It's satisfying. Those make for pretty good shifts. And when you get out on time. That's a really good shift.

The passage helps illustrate the purpose at the ED for many: identify something and fix it. The process of identification, then, becomes a way of understanding what quality care means within the ED. It's satisfying to be able to fix something and less so to manage chronic disease. Even more, the beginning is interesting in that good days come less from making a difference for patients and more about having food and playing jokes on each other.

In some ways, both seem to help providers cope or distract them from the complexities of the ED. Further yet, describing a good day by being able to see patients that can be fixed produces and organizes a type of care that finds quality in identifying, fixing, and moving on. Later on, this same provider describes a good shift by stating, "when you can intermingle with your colleagues…and maybe you saved a life or may be you made a big difference in a family with a patient." Both fixing and saving are practices embedded within the organization of the ED. And therefore, all care is directed towards practices that identify, treat, fix, and save. Another task in line with providing quality care is bringing situations that seem out of control, into control. For example, another nurse describes a good shift by saying,

> It's always a great day when you feel like you've helped somebody. When they come in in crisis and they leave and they've had something resolved, and they feel good. Or they have tools to go home with, so that they don't have to come here and utilize us as their primary source.

Resolving something is similar to fixing something in the ED, and both are satisfying. The satisfaction comes from the way the ED is organized towards a specific model of care where quality is understood a particular way. Part of the challenge, however, is managing providers' own energy and the energies of other patients. One doctor describes this as:

> There are people with their energies, they tend to dump it on you or they tend to take it out on you. And you are feeling pretty tired and worn out carrying all that energy around all day and I think it is learning how to manage yourself with that as your working environment.

It is important to mention that not only do providers feel stretched to manage patients, colleagues, and their own energy, but to manage them within other constraints like time can be overwhelming. One nurse described this challenge by saying,

> Time management becomes an issue. When you're so overworked and then you feel like you can never get caught up. I have that feeling of if my charting doesn't look right, my patients don't look right, everything kind of snowballs and it makes for a really long tiresome day and the patients end up suffering and so do I. You kind of see everything around just kind of fall apart.

The snowball effect does indeed make for a long tiresome day. Even more, in the ED, the use of protocols, time constraints, and standards moves things along at a constant and routine pace. But we know life doesn't quite work on standards, protocols, routines, and checklists. Providers must see anyone who walks through the door. As one nurse was told after complaining that a few patients had come in, "they're here, they're gonna get seen. Check 'em in and be nice. It's not gonna matter whether you like it or not, they're already here and they're gonna be seen."

This is standard thinking in the ED, just as it is standard to think quality care translates to providing care that can fix, save, or resolve a situation. These standards, however, are not terribly useful for dealing with complex patients and families who need more time to process their experience. These standards seem to help providers but bury some of the challenges of working here. Even more, rules, routines and protocols help to organize care and bring order to the rather un-orderly world of the ED. They also seem to bring some coherence to providers during rather incoherent situations as they walk a fine line between quantity and quality of care.

Even more, you can feel the challenges of providers feeling pulled to stay within the routine because it is expected of them and it is orderly. But you can also feel how they are pulled to make a difference in the medical care they provide. This environment produces a rhythm that is all-consuming. It is a rhythm that also helps bury some of the emotions, fears, wishes, and frustrations of working here. It is a rhythm that moves and steadies to the beats, buzzes, bells, and pages in the ED. In essence, it is a rhythm that helps to bring things under control. It helps to tame some of the more difficult and wild circumstances that come with working in the ED, like patients who are dying.

Following is a description of the final way providers manage the tension in the ED of feeling caught between rehumanizing care practices and providing quality care in an environment that wants to be fixed, saved, and resolved. It is no surprise, then, that the meaning and handling of death in the ED mirror the way care is organized and practiced.

Taming Death

The ED environment makes certain behaviors acceptable, like sarcasm. And around death, it is not only acceptable, but expected, to leave the room messy to illustrate that everything has been done to save the patient. In interviews, providers describe death in the ED as chaotic. As shown in my own crisis chapter, I experienced it this way also. But providers do some things that bring some control to their own work experiences. For example, one way of taming death can be felt through the following perception of what it means to be an ED physician:

> It's like a job like everybody else's job. You know you pack your lunch, go in hoping you get a few minutes to eat in peace. I mean, it's just weird, like I know you witnessed it but sometimes a patient will die and a minute later we are ordering pizza and it's not that we have disregard for that person's life, it's that—that's our job and it's no different than the guy who is a car mechanic who it is tragic for the car owner whose transmission fell out, who can't afford to replace it and that car is dead. Yeah, you say, we're talking about a life. I get that but everything is still a job to you and you don't want us to be—I mean what are you going to do, somebody dies in the ER and everyone has to go home because they are so emotionally distraught so we have to bring in a whole new crew?

In some ways, this passage underscores how the use of protocols and time constraints help bring order to this environment and the care it provides. It's a job, she says, and it's no different from someone else's. This reframing of what it means to work in the ED as something not exceptional and incredibly courageous, as I think, but rather something ordinary, shapes how care is delivered, especially around death.

Even more, having to bring in a whole new crew organizes the role and place of emotions as something separate from this experience. Knowing that emotions are not accepted or tolerated requires that providers think of their work in a way that helps prevent them from being totally emotionally distraught. Even more, thinking this way makes ordering pizza a logical decision, as opposed to something else that might not keep life coherent and orderly. One nurse describes how dying in the ED is better here:

> It's much better here in the hospital 'cause you know in the ER you treat them, you get them stable and you move them on. Or you know sometimes unfortunately they die but you know you've done your best and you've worked really hard on them.

The language in this passage, that providers "worked really hard" on patients, could seem difficult, if not offensive, to hear. But this language fits the ED; it is their purpose. And it also helps to tame a process like death, which is very complex. This is what they have been trained to do and what we expect them to do. Providers even mention how time and workload can interfere with caring for people who are dying; as one nurse said, "I think we sometimes have to find the time, even if it's for five minutes or taking them to a quiet room." Seconds later, she states "death is a hard thing for most people." It is especially hard because of the many interests invested into care practices at the end of life.

With that said, let me share a few stories that will help you feel some of the tensions and challenges of caring for people whose interests, as well as the interests of the organization and system, don't align with providers or patients. Kelly, a nurse in the ED who at the time was working in labor and delivery, shared a story with me about how the department didn't allow recently-born babies to be with their parents when they were dying because,

> We just took 'em. They didn't let parents hold them while they were dying. And there was one day that we were so busy, so busy. I mean we must have had 20 babies in one shift. And that's a lot for labor and delivery. And we had a pre-termer that was too young to save, and I kind of put 'em over aside, like we needed the room, so I couldn't even leave him in the room. Like I had to put him on a table in the sterile equipment thing. And I'm running around and I walk past the room and I happen to catch him, and I saw him breathing. And I was like, 'God, I let him die cold.'

This example sensitively illustrates how difficult it is to provide individual care within a fast paced and complex system. But acting otherwise in a system organized around rules, routines, checklists, and protocols is difficult. This same nurse went on to share another story about a baby who was "deformed"; another nurse told her that a pregnant colleague didn't want to touch this baby or "have anything to do with her." Kelly, however, said,

> 'Let me take care of this baby.' And I held that baby because like I said to God, I was not going to let anybody die like that again. I wrapped her up, I put a hat on her, and I fed her. They [colleagues] didn't want me to feed her. And I told the doctor, I said, 'you know, I can do a lot of things. I understand what's happening with this baby, but I'm not going to starve this baby to death. There's plenty of other things that are going to kill this baby, and me not feeding her is not one of 'em. 'Cause she's crying to be fed, she's hungry. She's going to get fed. Now you can turn your back and you can walk away and you cannot look at it, but this child will be fed. Period.'

I share both of these examples to help you experience some of the challenges, especially around death, that unfold when organizational norms intersect with humanistic norms. Just like patients, providers' experiences with death help to shape their attitudes towards it. Even more, organizational and institutional norms help shape attitudes and practices, just like at hospice and in the ED. The first example shared by Kelly begins with describing how busy the department was that day, similar to the ED, where the need to try to find room for patients, even placing patients on stretchers in the halls, is common as the waiting room and ambulance arrivals are persistent.

You can imagine the messiness of labor and delivery, with screaming babies being placed on cold metal tables and people moving fast. And you can also imagine the incoherence and struggle for Kelly to feed the baby that no one wanted to handle in the second example. The standard is to identify, fix, and move patients along, even at the end of life. These standards, however, play an intriguing role around death and dying.

A room in the ED after a patient has died or "coded" is a mess, literally. But this is common, expected, and in line with the purpose of care in the ED. Even more, to get a feel for what it is like to see someone die in the ED, take the following example, where a nurse describes how the family is often inside the room while providers try to save a patient's life:

> Before it was like get them out of the room, we need to do our job. And now it's like, leave them in the room. And I think if it were my kid I'd want to be in the room. But I know enough not to interfere, even as a nurse. But that poor person assigned to me is going, 'why are they doing that? What about this? Can't they do that? Did they get the magnesium?!' And I think we're really sensitive to that, and you get to a point where you just do anything 'cause they're, you know, they're dead, and maybe the magnesium will help. And if the family member wants two amps of magnesium pushed and that will help with their closure, that they felt like they interjected and they got to see everything done, then why not?

The ED rooms, where the patient and family stay, are messy according to one nurse because,

> We clean the blood off their face, but we leave all the tubes and everything. And we don't clean the rooms anymore. Like it used to be clean up the room, tuck 'em into bed, make 'em look like they're sleeping. Now it's like leave the crap everywhere so that they know that we opened the core cart—we went through all this equipment trying to save your family member. You know, and there's some, I don't know if it's research or just a person's theory, but there's an emerging theory that says that family members feel comforted when they see the room a mess.

Providers leave all the "crap" everywhere that was used to save a life so the family knows that they "opened the core cart." Without such evidence and stuff thrown everywhere, many families don't believe providers did all that they could.

Life in the ED is disorderly, just as death is. Keeping death messy and chaotic, however, is a way of taming death within the ED. The story at the

beginning of this chapter helped you get a feeling for the intricate balance
that is walked between institutional and humanistic norms within the ED.
Even more, the subsequent examples of providers' experience were introduced
for you to get a feeling for not only what it's like working here, but also how
providers do work here every day. And clearly, it takes work to do so, whether
it is transforming care practices that are organized by protocols, standards,
and routines, or thinking of their job just like any other job. In doing so, these
practices help illustrate the enormous tensions felt inside the ED as providers bear witness to heavy stories, experiences, and feelings. And yet they are
expected to handle these heavy stories, experiences, and feelings in much
the same way as they deliver care: through protocols, standards, routines, and
checklists.

We turn to emergency medical care when our ills are severe and not so severe because we know someone will care for us no matter what, when, where.
In short, we expect much of emergency providers, but too few of us ever wonder what it is like to have God-like surgical powers, yet to struggle against
your own humanity. What is it like to try and save a life, then be paged to tell
someone they have a terminal diagnosis, before being paged again to go see
a patient with a laceration from a wine glass? As individuals enter EDs with
many differing expectations, emergency medicine is driven by the need to
help others where they can.

ED patients have endless motivations for going there. Many come more
for reassurance, many come for information, many come to be comforted, and
many come for hope. Patients in the ED rely heavily on words, and often these
words are used for specific purposes. Words become the way hope, despair, fear,
medicine, cure, and care are created. Words like "there is nothing we can do
for you"; "your liver is going to fail if you continue drinking"; "your husband is
an alcoholic and you need to be careful because this a very long and difficult
path you are about to go on"; "No, I don't think you are going to die but you
have a very serious illness that needs to be taken care of properly or else maybe
you could die"; "we need to admit your son to the hospital because his HIV
has gotten more aggressive"; or "you have seven brain tumors" are not easily
spoken.

These words carry weight and these words certainly challenge our assumptions and expectations of medicine and care. And these words are difficult at
best when the goal is not only to care for patients but also give patients and
families at some vision that this isn't a hopeless and helpless situation. We
expect the ED to treat each of our unique ailments while expecting those

who are providing care to be quick, competent, intelligent, hopeful, and compassionate. But they, too, have their own fears of getting ill. And they, too, experience bad days, have problems with family and romantic partners and get tired and sick.

In the ED, like in the hospice, questions about illness and health and, to a lesser extent, life and death dance together intimately. A set of tensions seems to be organizing care in both settings to help refashion care practices in a way that brings some control to the disorder and incoherence that beats and breathes at each site. Although these tensions surrounding providing humanistic care within institutional norms take different forms, their goal—to—tame death remains the same. What is interesting, of course, is how taming becomes part strategic, part routine, and part improvisational for understanding the meaning of death and also life. The purpose of this project is not to argue that the way these places are organized is inherently wrong. Rather, my purpose has been to show and tell the stark difficulties of these places. The stories of providers at both the ED and hospice need to be told, for in them, we all must wonder—is this the best we can do at the end of life?

These ideas will be developed further and I will describe how the way death is being produced at both places enables and constrains critical understandings surrounding care practices. The next chapter will also describe how managing these tensions makes working in their presence easier, while making others more difficult, like supporting and hearing the voices, stories, and fears of the patients, families, and providers behind the double-glass doors at both sites. And finally, I will address why accepting a system that embraces chaos is so difficult to do, but also what would be needed for both places to accept a system that lives with chaos instead of always trying to manage and suppress it.

· 7 ·

THE CONCEALING AND REVEALING
NATURE OF LANGUAGE

The last two chapters described how both the ED and hospice are experienced and understood by the providers who work there. They detailed the tension of providing humanistic care within and against institutional norms. And finally, the chapters developed three specific ways providers overcome this tension that when practiced together, ultimately tame a process that would otherwise be wild, chaotic, and uncertain. Through taming, however, providers are doing more than rehumanizing their care practices; they are actively producing meanings surrounding death that define how we can and should understand death within the ED and hospice. Therefore, the role of this chapter is twofold. First, I will describe how our understandings of death are formed through the accounts and stories of providers. Second, I will outline how in producing and defining meanings surrounding death, providers' talk is simultaneously enabling them to smooth over the complexities of their work while at the same time, talking in a language that protects them from critical engagement.

There is an inherent tension at the ED and the hospice. On the one hand, their purposes demand that they be routine, standardized, and efficient. And on the other hand, their role is to heal and provide humanitarian care in a demanding and chaotic setting. Embedded in these contradictions, however, are a number of suppressed conflicts and opportunities. Therefore, rather than simply showing you how providers manage their challenges, I will describe what these practices are doing. In order to detail what providers' talk and practices for taming death are doing for the meanings surrounding death, I will return to Gerry and Susan's narratives from Chapter One. A return to the narratives is also a return to the role of language and discourse in the production of death. But first, let me say a few things about language and discourse.

Providers at hospice and the ED use their creativity to deal with the messiness of both places. Listening to their stories and accounts from the previous chapters emphasizes that their stories need to be told and listened to. In doing so, we realize they are saying much about how death is handled and should continue to be handled. Yet their stories and accounts about death have implications for the meaning of death. Providers are very creative in handling death and at times work to decorate death as something unique, hard to understand without being there, and very difficult. But their attempts at decorating death or caretaking in general conceal conflicts and therefore suppress meanings from being contested around death.

Conflicts become suppressed in a variety of ways, especially around death. One conflict being suppressed is trying to make a difference in medical care embedded in a system that is remarkably routine. But this conflict becomes concealed through their language promoting the concept that life in the ED and the hospice is different from any other place. Even more, this conflict becomes suppressed through stories they choose to tell that reaffirm, if not naturalize for them, that what they are doing is special, different, and unique. These moves further suppress the ability for anyone to critically engage what it is like to work at these places.

For example, at the beginning of this book I discussed how many believe that the U.S. is a death-denying society. Through providers' accounts and stories, however, it is clear that we are not necessarily death-denying, but we are indeed fearful of death. Earlier I wrote about my unspoken anxieties about dying, even the possibility of dying, or someone close to me dying. When we fear, as I argue providers do, like me, we often stigmatize and shun death, and sometimes even try to deny the very possibility of death.

The first narrative, if you remember, comes from Gerry, a nurse practitioner at hospice. And recall that I have taken these passages from an interview with her; my questions are in bold font and her words in italics.

Consequences of Talk at Hospice

What's a bad day here? *Well a bad day is when I can't help somebody in the sense that they don't seem to understand what I am saying or maybe the team isn't able to communicate effectively—I mean that is really one of the key challenges with our role is what we say and what people hear.* This passage details the way the hospice begins to construct a particular meaning and a particular experience about death. Defining a bad day as when patients don't understand providers positions us to accept and prioritize that the providers' understanding must be prioritized. Imagine if a bad day were defined by feeling frustrated that providers couldn't understand patients. This would immediately prioritize a different kind of experience. Further, communication is understood through its effectiveness in communicating a message to the patient that they are not hearing in a way the hospice wants them to. The patient here is essentially being called out for not being able to understand "effectively" why they are at hospice. Imagine for a moment the perspective of the patient who just arrived at hospice after receiving a terminal diagnosis with not much time left to live. Further, imagine you've been admitted to a place that has quickly been defined as your new home, with few of your belongings and unfamiliar surroundings. And imagine what it would be like to hear that this is a place different from any other hospital setting you have been to as you stare out the window at the empty bird feeder, lying in a white sheet in an uncomfortable bed. Would you feel understood? For the patient, this might be one of the key challenges of coming to hospice, not feeling understood and not wanting their experience to be defined so quickly for them.

And if we are speaking different languages, which can often happen at the end of life, then poor communication is going to make for a really bad day. And it happens in all different shapes and sizes. Each situation is going to be different but if you have a day where you are just not able to communicate openly with another person, it's going to make for a really bad day. **What do you mean by different languages?** *Could be a cultural difference. Could be just a knowledge deficit about their disease process. It could be in the form of—maybe they are just in a different place of their illness, their journey—they might have an expectation that is not aligned with hospice necessarily. Not everyone comes to hospice knowing what hospice is or understanding what hospice is, or being ready for hospice. So we're not here, I'm not here to make them ready but to meet them where they're at and to see how I can help them best. And that may be staying here in hospice or it may be finding what's in line with their particular goals and values.*

The paragraph begins to decipher the way language is strategically used and how everyday terms shape interaction norms. Furthermore, everyday terms describing what hospice does, are often clarified by describing what it does not do. For the most part, what is identified in this paragraph are external constraints like, "different place of their illness," or "not everyone comes to hospice knowing what hospice is." Even more, we hear a unifying and colonizing voice speaking about hospice in general terms, not in specific terms about a particular setting. Further, medicine here comes across as having choices or "meeting them where they're at," but the options of "staying here in hospice" or "finding what's in line with their particular goals" leaves out a plethora of other options or alternatives. It is as if there is a variety of choice, but in actuality, it is more like an illusion of choice around end of life. Further, this paragraph already presumes a hospice frame: that "place" at hospice matters. The last sentence doesn't explicitly say options, but Gerry's language already frames a particular understanding that there are options for patients.

This enables her to explain how hospice is a unique environment. In essence, she is producing a difference for why people come. She never describes what the difference is but more importantly, in asserting they are different closes off examination and discussion. Additionally, Gerry refers to these as different languages, which has implications for how we understand communication at hospice. She states how speaking different languages often happens at the end of life as if to excuse, if not conceal, what some of the differences are. And stating that this "often happens," she begins to naturalize this understanding rather than leaving it open to critical engagement.

Feeling misunderstood, for both provider and patient, becomes understood as speaking different languages at the end of life. But actually, it is less "different languages" and more of a difference in the implicit values and beliefs of both patients and providers about what a fair death would look like, for example, and what providers' role is. Finally, calling these "different" languages underscores a dominant theme throughout hospice, that things are different and unique, including the language around life and death. Consequently, defining languages as being different closes off discussion or examination and instead begins to normalize and naturalize a belief that different languages really do develop at the end of life, thereby keeping them unquestioned.

What's important for this kind of work? *First and foremost, you are a human being so don't forget you are a human being! You have to be genuine. I would say listen to other people as much as you can and when you find that you are not* *able to interact with people anymore whether it is on that given day or that you have to take care of yourself or you're never going to be able to take care of other people. So care for yourself, be genuine.*

What is produced here is a fascinating orientation towards death that is about "being who you are" as if nothing else could matter. Embedded in the talk, however, is a push for authenticity and genuine interaction that includes moments that point to the difficulty of this work. For example, "as much as you can and when you find that you are not able to interact with people anymore" defines limits. Caring for the self becomes just as important as caring for other people. But telling people to be genuine is in reference to knowing that you are a human being that has limits and you should not forget that. It is as if her use of language is trying to infuse a sense of humanity into this work that tends to strip away in this unique environment, while reminding us all of our inherent limits as human beings. We miss critical important information about working here when it is described like this.

You have to be really empathetic. You have to be very compassionate. You absolutely have to have a good heart, which probably encompasses all of the above. I would say the primary characteristic that you really need is to be an empathetic person. But at the same time you have to realize that this is the patient's and family's experience and not your experience. So that they—the patient and the family—are essentially the ones that are going through this and you are trying to guide them.

To say someone needs characteristics of empathy and compassion, demands vulnerability. Even more, mentioning these qualities orients us to think of hospice as truly kindhearted. But interestingly, the next move, to remind someone that this is not their experience, is complicated because after all, it is difficult to be empathetic without somehow becoming part of another's experience. Empathy demands a sense of being part of something or someone other and asks people to feel, suffer, and celebrate similarly. It is a coming together to feel, suffer, and celebrate in a similar way. Providers are involved in this experience, too. But here providers are guides in the dying process, not players involved in the experience. They are guiding patients to a particular feeling and experience of end of life. And when they cannot, or when patients become resistant to accept this experience, providers describe this as a bad day or a frustration because of the different languages at end of life. When patients resist this experience, providers push back, feel that they aren't communicating "effectively," and this makes for a crummy shift. Because when patients resist, responsibility shifts away from a routine hospice death and other figures, including religious figures, take over. When patients resist, providers begin to feel as though they are not in control of someone's death unless they can communicate in a way where patients "buy in" to this way of dying.

Are there any barriers that get in the way trying to guide patients and families? *Yes, in fact, the day-to-day nonsense I like to call it, just the interruptions, the flow of events, and the work environment. Essentially, when I talk or meet with a patient and the family, I try to immerse myself in that experience and really close everything else out and not be thinking about what else I could be doing whether it's with another patient or whether it is something personal, to really give 100% when I am with that patient.*

Recall, however, that Gerry just reminded us that we are human beings with our own limits and to not forget that. But here, she describes how she tries to get close and immerse herself. Similarly, she just described how important it is to be empathetic but to know that this is not your experience, but the patients' and families'. Here, she is telling us again how important it is to be 100% present. These past few passages underscore glimpses of the difficulty of working here. Hospice promotes empathy and promotes life and living, which is why Gerry oscillates, coming back to the mission of hospice while also exposing what happens when patients resist this particular experience. Even more, interruptions become barriers because in many ways, they disrupt the routine ways of caretaking, if not even dislodging providers' ability to think for a moment about something different.

Further, the way Gerry describes her patient experiences with language like "immersion," "empathy," "close everything else out," and "give 100%," attempts to define a hospice experience as something different where these activities are normal. But how can we begin to talk about the dying experience at hospice when each experience is so unique and special and "heavy"? We can't. Because these experiences become defined as so deeply personal and authentic that it prevents any one from talking about these experiences in any way other than the way hospice is doing.

Being a nurse to me is something really special. It is something that is very personal, it's just a very unique relationship that you have with another individual that you aren't always able to share in other locations or professions. And it's something that, being a nurse to me it's more about, it's not just the medical piece or the health piece—it's really relating to that person in a way where they feel open enough to disclose things that are very personal and private issues. And you have to earn their trust, you have to earn their relationship, you have to know just because I am a nurse doesn't mean you have to tell me everything about you.

Working here is something to be proud of because it is a way of relating to someone in a particular way. Her description of what it means to be a nurse describes a rather prestigious and sacred profession. Not everyone experiences this extraordinary relationship. There is something sacred about it that is not "able to share in other locations or professions." Further, she describes being a nurse as something more than the medical role in the relational qualities of healing professions. They are in a particular relationship with someone in which medical care is delivered by a special, humanitarian professional. If you believe in this philosophy, it supposedly will guide you to some place better around end of life.

Are there specific things that you do with patients? *Yes, of course. I try to just get to know the person. It's hard because there is a blur between personal and professional but I just try and engage the individual just talking with them, not just coming in and just focusing on the issue at hand. I mean if I come in and say how is your breathing today? If that is going to be the extent of my relationship with a person, then that is probably how they are going to disclose things to me, reveal things to me and that's all our relationship is going to be. For hospice, where we all wear multiple hats and even though I assume the medical provider/nursing piece of their care, I can't shut them down if they want to talk about something else because that is not what it is all about. So I essentially just try and get to know that person, try to get to know what they are comfortable revealing to me and go from there. Hospice care is difficult and people often don't have a good sense of what it is.* **How come?** *Well, there is a real interest coupled with fear. It's a real conversation stopper at times. There are a lot of people that just say, "oooohhhh." My family and friends will still ask me but there is still kind of a veil that comes over them when they talk with me about how are things at hospice, their voice changes and it's serious stuff and I realize in conversation with them how open I have become to talking about dying and the end of life and how comfortable I am on a professional level with discussing dying and end of life issues.* **Do they understand what you really do?** *A lot of times, for example, my family and friends will ask me exactly what I do and they have an accurate impression. My brother, he doesn't live in town and he has known that I have worked as a nurse practitioner at hospice and he kind of skirts the issue a little bit. You know I don't think he fully understands what I do.*

Hospice as a "conversation stopper" is not surprising. Just the words can close communication because they mean something strong, yet mysterious to so many of us. But why can't we talk about hospice like providers do? Gerry mentions how "comfortable" she has become talking about death but there seems to be a disconnect with what providers say and what patients (and I) experience. Her talk immediately tames the seriousness of how people's voices change when she mentions she works at hospice. Talk at hospice tries to produce a different kind of death that often runs in direct opposition to the dominant discourses surrounding the place, its smell, its philosophy, and its name. But the place, the smell, and its philosophy of care become concealed or closed off through the tremendous work their language is doing to produce such a unique experience at the end of life that providers, patients, and families begin to take on as their own, without question. Gerry mentions how comfortable she has become talking about death.

Habits are comfortable, just like talking about something in a particular way for so long becomes comfortable. Feeling comfortable talking about death begins to sensitize even the surroundings of the place. But these surroundings, to any "naked eye" or un-socialized eye, are tremendously visible and difficult not to see. Language conceals these things from not only being seen, but from being critically examined, because the values embedded in hospice about life, living, and authenticity take priority, thereby making certain meanings visible and believable and not others.

Why do you think this problem exists? *I think a lot of it is very emotionally charged. You know each and every one of us has known someone who has died and for most people it kind of elicits a painful emotion, probably a mixture of feelings. And so when people talk about dying, especially if they don't have the professional perspective, it becomes a very personal event and it's kind of, they may be respectful, they may feel a lot of gratitude towards hospice professionals in the past but for a lot of people it really isn't a pleasant experience so it is something that makes them very emotional and not necessarily in a good way.*

Professionalism here is intriguing, because for her it makes reality easier to accept, rather than allowing it to become "a very personal event." But death is personal and unique! Her talk almost disregards feelings and emotions at the end of life that make it an unpleasant experience. What's even more interesting is how having "the professional perspective" is producing a new meaning of professionalism that embodies being in relation, fully immersed, taking care of yourself, and just trying to get to know the person. She says how non-professional people talk about death as a personal event. This illustrates how hospice does not avoid death, but is an interesting plethora of competing voices about death. Their talk sets up the incredible difficulty of working here, and the real pleasures of working here. More, this kind of talk works to humanize who they are and how they identify themselves during a dehumanizing experience. We hear incoherent, contradictory voices about death and hospice that begin to leave us all at a standstill, wanting to examine them because what we often thought death to be is being defined for us differently.

This short narrative exposes an interesting way of packaging death and putting aside meanings that compete with the philosophy of hospice. Even more, this packaging of death gives us glimpses of the real difficulty of this place and the real difficulty of this work. We hear distinct calls to the sacredness of their professions, but wonder whether they are still sacred in an environment that is remarkably routine even though its narrative tries to make it not routine. Consequently, providers seek to transform what otherwise would be routine through language that, for the most part, is sealed off to others who have not seen, felt, and heard what their world is like. More specifically, the packaging of death becomes a way to code language surrounding death. Essentially, this coded language produces a space of taboo talk. It is not that death is not talked about, but rather death is talked about in a very unusual and coded way that tries to make the "non-beautiful" parts of death, invisible.

For example, hospice workers code death through their language use around empathy and authenticity that shapes a particular meaning about caretaking. And the ED workers code death through their use of language that asserts that no one can understand the ED without being there. Consequently, this coded language becomes accepted and habitual, closing itself off from critical examination. In short, coding language around death makes it so no one, in fact, has to face the fear of death; through coded language we have essentially worked to stigmatize dying experiences as being nothing but routine.

Consequences of Talk at the ED

Interestingly, these same moves and consequences of talk are not unique to hospice, they also infuse the ED. Let's now return to the earlier narrative in Chapter One from Susan, an ED physician. Again, I will go paragraph by paragraph to describe not just what she is saying, but what is being done.

It's like a job like everyone else's job. You know you pack your lunch, hoping you get a few minutes to eat in peace. I mean, it's just weird, you know sometimes a patient will die and a minute later we are ordering pizza and it's not that we have disregard for that person's life, it's that—that's our job and it's no different from the guy who is a car mechanic where it is tragic for the car owner whose transmission fell out, who can't afford to replace it and that car is dead. Yeah, you say, but we're talking about a life. I get that but everything is still a job and you don't want us—I mean what are you going to do, someone dies in the ER and everyone has to go home because they are so emotionally distraught so we have to bring in a whole new crew? That is a hard thing for people to get. It's not that we are not compassionate—we've been doing it for 20 years and our job goes on. As soon as you finish with this one person who died and console their family, now you are 15 people behind and they are all mad as hell at you.

Comparing her job to that of a car mechanic informs our understanding of the ED. For one, it immediately transforms the place into something normative and instrumental: this is a job with routines that we follow. As soon as you finish, you have 15 people behind and they are all mad as hell. This sounds like an uncomfortable place to work. Further, she goes on to ask whether we expect them to bring in a whole new crew after someone died because they are so emotionally distraught. In so doing, her language tries to normalize work and life in the ED. She "packs her lunch" and "hopes to get a few minutes to eat in peace." But we know ED providers talk much about the mystery and uniqueness of the place, but, like the hospice, it is still a job.

Even though they are dealing with individual lives, it is still a job. The implication of referring to it as just a job provides a glimpse into the real routineness of their work. Even more, the moment that glimpse becomes visible she follows with a statement that asserts again they are different. It is hard to imagine a situation where everyone would be so emotionally distraught that they would call in a whole new crew. But in saying this, she closes off examination of her job because after all, she is dealing with a life, not a car. More, her language pulls you near in a way that makes you feel bad for providers. But the moment you get sucked into their thoughts and feelings, as I did, is also the moment critical examination stops and things become accepted rather than questioned.

What makes for a good day at work? *I think the personalities in the ER—different nurses, and other docs you are working with—is definitely one of the bigger variables. If you've got the right mix, everyone has good energy, it's funny, sarcastic, playful, and we can diffuse a patent's energy with each other. The patients that wear us down are the patients that are demanding, have ridiculous expectations, like I have had this for fifteen years and I have seen 10 specialists and I am here Friday night at 10 pm and I expect you to have an answer to why this is going on. That can be absurd and sometimes you can let it roll off you but sometimes patients are so in your face and make you in your weak moments really defensive and engage that behavior and that makes for a bad shift.*

Here you can feel how providers let things "roll off" and find energy in each other in order to cope. Even more, you pick up on the real changes of this place. The way it is said comes out as a struggle and you can even feel a sense of the difficulty in this work. She sounds worn out when she talks about how patients wear them down. Finding play and fun in other colleagues to diffuse a patient's energy reminds you of the struggle within this talk, and therefore the struggle of this work.

And then there are other things in the mix that make for a bad shift—last night it was a bad shift because there were a lot of patients that had a lot of sad diagnoses, like one woman came in, had breast cancer 15 years ago, she had bilateral mastectomies, they didn't recommend chemo and radiation, they said it was not called for it was such a small tumor and she comes in with a complaint of a herniated disc kind of symptoms and has enough neurological symptoms that I did an MRI because she had lost her reflex, she had lost some bladder control, and sometimes that means you have to do something surgical. Got an MRI and she had boney metastases throughout…and you know it was like taking all the wind out of her sail and I think she thought it was never something she'd ever worry about that came back…you know that is hard, it's hard to give somebody that diagnosis, it's hard to feel like in the ER you're doing anything but dumping all this horrible information on them saying, alright, why don't you follow up with your doctor, we need the bed, there's 15 more in the waiting room.

Again, it sounds like someone just took the wind out of her sail. Describing how the process of giving bad news is tough in the ED, and you feel in her voice how much this work is getting to her. You can feel a sense of struggle in trying to help and do something different in a system that continuously dumps bad information on people. It is as though the difficulty of this kind of work sucks the energy out of these professionals and the difference they are able to make in our care and health.

You know it's like you can't spend enough time with them—you know it's not like they need you to spend more time with them that minute because they need some time to take it all in and sort it out, but the ER seems like a funny place to be handing out that info. So, bad diagnoses can wear us down because we are people too you know and we have our own illness and fears about getting illnesses or it might remind you of a friend you had that had something and it just sometimes gets really personal and it's hard to keep up your defenses and it's not to say that you are like a wall and impervious to all that is around you but I don't know that people get that. At some level we have to have the wall up or we would be consumed by horrific diagnoses and sadness and other stuff we do.

What is interesting here is how the everyday terms identify internal constraints like, "bad diagnoses can wear us down," or "we have our own illness and fears about getting illnesses." Furthermore, the notion of "place" is interesting here like, "the ER seems like a funny place to be handing out that info." The physical place of the ER becomes its own norm or way to organize what and how things can be discussed and not discussed. Also, language here includes unifying terms such as "we are people too." Because the framing is turned inwards onto the self, medicine takes an interesting role as people are putting up "defenses" in order to not be "consumed" by "horrific diagnoses" and "sadness." In other words, these interaction norms point to the work that medicine and physical space demand of individuals, thereby highlighting other underlying logics at play. These terms carry inherent ideological properties, like the physical place of the emergency department that organizes how care is administered. Even more, the ideological properties of place help organize emergency medicine's own set of tensions, strategies, and protocols for how to accomplish the work with the language being used. Her language simultaneously distinguishes what is acceptable and not in the ED.

Having to try and save someone's life while family are wailing right next to you, is not an easy task. You have to somewhere put it aside and though you know it hurts—you're trying to help somebody and I guess that is the hardest part that in medicine, at some point you have to figure out how to manage it and if you don't find a way to let it out later it starts to make you a bitter, cynical, burned out doctor that takes it out on people and that is the end result that patients see and say what an ass that doc is, but they might not appreciate all the pain and suffering we've had to bear witness to that has taken its toll on us, even though we signed up for it. It still is hard and they don't teach us how to manage that. And there are conferences and lectures on how to handle the difficult patient or whatever but it is not really something we embrace. You know it's not like, hey look what I am going to. It's more you take it on because somewhere down the line you learn you've got to do these things to save yourself.

Reading this you can imagine just how much pain and suffering she and others have had to witness. Have providers always experienced so much pain and suffering? Her language highlights how life in the ED feels like they only give interventional treatment before moving on to the next patient. But her talk also underscores how she wishes care could be different. That is, how it could be more faithful, honest, and sacred. In short, she does a beautiful job of producing and defining meanings surrounding how death is handled in the ED.

The language used by both Gerry and Susan produces particular experiences of the way death is handled. Further, their talk enables them to smooth over the complexities of working while at the same time, talking in a language that protects them and their work from critical engagement. The latter is where I will turn to next.

The first part of this chapter has focused on what language enables providers to do around end of life. This part will focus on how the same language closes off their work practices and experiences from critical engagement. In doing so, important conflicts are being suppressed and lost surrounding how meaning is being produced at the end of life and how different choices might become thinkable.

The last chapters have illustrated how providers produce a particular experience for caretaking around the end of life. Part of understanding this experience is understanding how their worlds are organized around the tension of providing humanistic care in an environment that is uncomfortably regulated and routine. The tension for the most part is irresolvable, yet it is solved in some ways through the rehumanizing of care practices and even in the stories they have chosen to tell me. Why, for example, did the nurse tell me about saving a baby from dying cold on a metal table? Or why did the doctor at the ED choose to tell me the story about the couple from Europe and the laceration from the wine glass? Both of these stories happened months if not several years ago. Why are they still telling them? Why when asked about delivering bad news, did the doctor tell me this? And why, when asked about how they have been socialized to think about death, did the nurse tell me a story from several years ago about not wanting to let a baby die hungry or cold? The stories help them cope. They also help them justify their existence and give them meaning in a remarkably routine environment. These stories seem to be doing something further yet.

Providers solve this tension partially by suppressing a part of what they don't want to necessarily deal with: the out-of-control nature of death. The stories become one way of not having to face the complexity of death through the translation of narrative rationality to technical rationality. Even more, providers' language promoting that their organizations are different, unique, and hard to understand unless you are there becomes another way of not having to face death. And further yet, these moves illustrate how quickly stories, even complex stories, become understood through an actionable list. These moves, or activities that take place, serve as a blockage, thereby closing off opportunities for things to be done differently.

Discursive Closure at the End of Life

Committed to a critical and dialogic approach from the outset, this book is concerned with the way language and meaning become distorted. It is not enough to say that providers' practices tame death. Rather, I want to share what happens when death becomes tamed, and I want to share what happens when organizations endlessly produce the meaning that they are different and unique from others.

For the most part, I have been working with competing discourses of care. But embedded in society are also larger and more dominant discourses that promote an orientation toward life, that embrace living to the fullest, until we die. Similarly, these discourses promote saving and fixing a life at all costs, which has become routine, standardized, and naturalized. The ED and the hospice organize their practices around these discourses and are essentially being organized by these same discourses. From Chapter One, we know that discourses are ideological and infused with implicit values that prioritize what kinds of choices become thinkable, and which choices are made. And of course, a host of other values, other meanings, and other choices remains invisible.

Other values about how death should be handled, or where death should take place, or how much pain we are willing to bear get suppressed when language tames death. Providers do this too. By taming death, they are not simply mediating their experiences; rather they are actively suppressing something that becomes too much to stomach every day. In essence, taming death through language begins to shift some responsibility away from them to the purpose of the organization, that is, to save and embrace life until the very end. Even more, what is happening by transforming the uniqueness and complexity of death is that the meanings and practices surrounding death are being reproduced. In doing so, what is being suppressed and blocked is the unspokenness of the real fear of dying or getting ill.

The way death is handled, however, depends on the way language is being used, and our access to language. At the hospice and the ED, language is used to smooth over the complexity and difficulty of their work to make life easier. Their lives are routine at these sites even though the stories they choose to tell, and not tell, or the things they want you to see, and not see, become ways to expose the values embedded in their talk, their desire to think that it is something other than routine. Stories about seeing six people die, for example, or watching a hospice patient get married at their chapel, or sharing a story about telling a patient they have seven brain tumors, are all events that don't happen every day. Yet these stories serve as reminders that their work is different, important, and unique in an environment organized around protocols and routines.

Further, providers believe in their stories. I believed in them. They described them as if they just happened a few days ago. I felt them as if they happened every day. Stories blocked me from seeing things, however. And I imagine they block providers from seeing things as well. As a result, providers use these routines to not only tame death, but to hide behind the complexity of it. Think, for example, how often providers at both places promote that they are unique and different. What does this do for them?

Promoting that the ED and the hospice are different from other settings, and saying that you can't know what they are like until you have spent time there, immediately makes it so we can't talk about them. Claiming uniqueness seals them off from any really critical engagement. Spending time in these places, however, I quickly realized that there is nothing quite unique about either one, even though they continue to say they are different and that you have to be there to experience them or else you won't "get it." Even more, in claiming uniqueness, providers' experience becomes subjectified and also sealed off from critical engagement. No one is supposed to ever really be able to understand these places or providers outside dominant discourses that promote the role of providers as godlike figures with infinite power and knowledge.

Their experiences become understood as so deeply personal and painful that no one believes they can ask about or understand them. But providers do talk. They freely tell stories that make people curious about them. They choose to share stories that make others impressed with their power, knowledge, and compassion in these environments.

Interestingly, the first few days I observed the ED I was taken up to the ICU to watch morning rounds. It was terribly uncomfortable and perhaps they wanted me to see and experience the real pain and suffering of these places to begin shaping everything I saw or heard. Similarly, when I first started observing the hospice, I was invited for three days in a row to "get the whole hospice experience." I was initiated, or disciplined, from the very start to orient myself towards seeing and feeling in a particular way about how death is handled in these settings. In short, I was learning the language and learning the code.

Further, by sealing their experiences and stories off from others, we all in a way are slowly stigmatizing these professions by not critically engaging them, their experiences, or the system in which they work. Claiming uniqueness seems to constrain all of our ability to talk with providers, discuss our options about death, and understand both more meaningfully.

Both places are producing and colonizing their own spaces of taboo talk about death. There is not silence around death but rather a river of voices speaking about death, albeit in ways that are coded. The coded nature of providers' talk becomes the very way they handle and organize the tension surrounding death. In trying to solve the tension of providing humanistic care in environments that are uncomfortably routine, providers speak in a language that is accessible, routine, and familiar to them.

Further, taming death allows providers to not face the wildness of death as it is believed to unfold. But what is happening is that providers are reproducing a very particular routine way of handling death at both the ED and the hospice. The handling of death is routine, thereby closing off a plethora of other choices that could be made. Even more, the routine ways of handling death are leaving much unspoken. The invisible and unspoken must be heard in order to bring some kind of contestation to meanings surrounding death so that stories do not become our only way of encountering difference in environments that suppress difference.

The values embedded in these routine choices are exposed through discourses and the ways they prioritize what kind of language to use, what behaviors are acceptable, what feelings are right, what choices are available, and what choices we should make around the end of life. Why, for example, don't people clap when someone dies at hospice? Part of the reason is because the value system defining death does not include celebrating the end of life. Rather, our values foster fighting and holding on until the very end. Why, for example, when I asked the doctor to share a time when she delivered bad news, didn't she say, "I had to tell an 18-year-old last night that her foot was broken and she'd be out for the soccer season?" In many ways, this would have produced a very different understanding of the ED, different from a story about telling someone they have a terminal disease.

Or what would it have done if, when I asked what made for a good day at hospice, a nurse had told me, "the moment that we can do something different and not follow a routine procedure"? Why, for example, don't providers say how happy and relieved they are when someone who had been suffering dies? Why don't providers share how frustrating and routine their days can be at the hospice or the ED and how difficult that becomes for their own relationships? And why, as patients, aren't we generally curious about these professions, how they cope, and how they wind down at the end of the day? In many ways, these questions remain unasked because the belief systems about death have no place for these questions that might cause different words, actions, and behaviors to become thinkable or take priority, or even to be chosen when caring for a patient at the end of life. Indeed, the discourse of preserving life is powerful.

· 8 ·

CONCLUSIONS, IMPLICATIONS, AND REFLECTIONS

This book explained how discourses influence and provide particular rhythms for understanding life and death. Even more, it described how competing discourses orient us to the world in a particular way and in so doing, put into play a way of feeling, thinking, and talking about death. Further, this book scrutinized how language organizes meaning and also naturalizes meaning around care, health, and death. Beyond organizing and naturalizing, however, this study illustrated how these discourses are decorated to be unique and different but are inherently chaotic, wild, and tension-filled, thereby putting into play competing relationships around end of life. In short, discourses around end of life are in crisis.

I use the word crisis not to define that our ways of responding to death are broken because, as I mentioned in Chapter One, that suggests there are ways to fix it. This is not the case. Rather, by crisis I mean a crisis over meaning and a crisis over what to value at the end of life. The good thing is that a crisis can be a turning point in a sequence of events (Treichler, 1990). Healthcare reform in many ways bespeaks of a society trying to figure out what to value. And what to value is largely determined by meanings surrounding health. This study has not judged health care practices, but looked at how dying patterns shed light on a larger system of meaning.

A crisis over meaning surrounding health care offers society and economies a turning point where the negotiation of meanings are contested even in subtle ways, questioning accepted practices and assumptions about dying. Again, the crisis is not about death, but about the meanings surrounding death. And both sites studied here have incredible power and access to produce, reinforce, and colonize a particular understanding of death and dying.

For example, producing meaning around death standardizes insurance rates and reimbursements for how death should be handled and where it should be handled. Further, meaning determines where providers must work and spend their time with patients. Even more, it standardizes what can be said around end of life and standardizes our access to resources around end of life. And, even more troubling, colonizing meaning standardizes specific smells, sounds, colors, and feelings around end of life. Clearly, our meanings and widely accepted practices and assumptions about death are colonizing and, even more, are in a constant flow in one direction. This kind of inertia is naturalizing certain behaviors and practices around death, even though they are also being disrupted.

Dying patterns are being disrupted on many levels including legislative battles, rising insurance costs, overcrowded waiting rooms, aging populations, increased chronic illnesses, battles over provider compensation, medical error, soaring healthcare costs, provider shortages, and social media. Importantly, this study has illustrated that these disruptions are largely played out in language. This study also informs us that we know that these same disruptions are filled with tensions and contradictions. In the pages of this book, we have felt the unforgettable rhythm of both of these sites that are subtly calling into question some of our widely accepted practices and assumptions about dying. This same rhythm has disturbed our current understandings of much of health communication research.

Adding to Our Health Care Understanding

This book moved beyond a mere description of the behaviors and practices in healthcare settings to illustrate the trenches of clinical life. It took Hirschmann's (1999) advice of going to the trenches and training grounds of clinical life, where lived experience unfolds. In doing so, it helps underscore the importance of context, culture, and language to understand what is going on and explain why this is going on. Further, it extended Hirschmann's call to develop evocative accounts that put pressure on health researchers today to develop more textured theories of communication and human interaction that respond to the changing field of medicine.

I did not intentionally try to make this book messy or complex, but these sites are messy and complex. For that reason, I believe dwelling on the disorder of life and human interaction rather than trying to "clean up the mess" allows us to experience a much more textured feeling of life in these environments. This textured feeling matters for health research because it conveys a sense of what these places are really like, how they are experienced, and how providers manage their own selves working in these settings. Even more, this feeling has introduced you to a host of norms, realities, stories, and experiences that are rarely heard and deeply misunderstood. After all, we learn best from and with others.

For that reason, this book respected the voices of others in generating knowledge with my decision to incorporate providers' as well as my own experiences of these places. Although the ways I have incorporated these voices and quotes are somewhat subjective, there is tremendous value in paying attention to the people who work in these settings. After all, providing a more evocative account through the voices of others around end of life has allowed me to detail the tension-filled nature of these places. My study moved beyond mere behavioral accounts of clinic life to the tensions and struggles of these sites. In doing so, this study has helped develop a richer understanding of interpersonal interaction to include the complexity and dynamics of these relationships that are being produced in a variety of competing ways. Providing accounts that better respond to our changing social situations, especially around death, is useful for developing models of communication that are more responsive to the endless tensions and struggles over meaning. Further, this study provided a contextualized understanding that has revealed how death is not orderly, static, and coherent, but is fragmented, full of paradoxes and ironies. After all, life is complicated, and so must be our understanding and theories of communication and interaction if we want to be able to respond and act meaningfully in a variety of settings.

More Useful Ways of Thinking and Talking

I did little at the time when I was observing the ED and the hospice to directly reflect on the ways in which providers understood and framed the tensions inherent in their jobs. It was not until I had left the field that I began to see and feel how different people come to make sense of contradictory meanings in different ways. I experienced contradictory meanings surrounding death at both places, which I wrote about earlier.

Providers at the ED and hospice, on the other hand, have particular and recurring ways for dealing with and resolving the tension around providing humanistic care in environments organized by institutional norms. Embedded in their talk are stunning contradictions that slowly begin to surface through their routine practices. For example, organizing providers' experiences around tensions allowed me to see how they enjoyed sharing their experience about how meaningful work is to them. But in practice, these wishes and hopes often got suppressed in an effort to provide care in light of organizational routine practices that stripped away some of their best and most honest intentions for making a difference in medical care. More, organizing providers' experience around tensions helped this study move away from individuals' behaviors to an understanding, and critique, of the social and organizational conditions under which individuals act in regard to medical care.

Even more, organizing their experiences around tensions exposed the complexities and contradictions of how a particular culture handles and constructs death. Exposing the complexities and contradictions of the way death is handled adds to our understanding of organizations and even more, to processes of organizing.

Specifically, this project illustrated how the ED and the hospice organize in the first place and continue to stay organized through a transformation of care practices that ultimately worked to tame death. Even more, this study adds to theories of discourse by describing what happens when discourses like those that surround the ED and the hospice become organized and disrupted.

Earlier in this project I identified several ways discourses have been understood and at the time, I thought they were very useful ways of making sense of discourses. But what is missing is an understanding of what happens when discourses compete and even more, how discourses become coded and closed off from critical engagement. The additions to our understanding of discourse are useful because they illustrate how old and often standardized models of care cannot always represent the complexity and extraordinary nature of human life. Further, understanding discourses as fleeting and competing allows for spaces to become visible where actual lived experience unfolds. These spaces detail how discourses become organized and disorganized, thereby making visible meanings that have previously been suppressed and unquestioned.

Focusing on discourses and the ways they become organized exposed the juxtaposition of these places. Even more, processes of disorganizing help to see and feel the emotional, performative, and unpredictable nature of this work. Further, this study and its attention to organizing features of talk did so from the sites where actual lived experience unfolded. For that reason, this study is unique in its practical contributions.

Practical Contributions

From the outset, the ED and hospice have asserted that they are unique and that you can't really understand what they are like until you are there. This focus on distinction allows both sites to claim uniqueness through their talk, care practices, behavior, stories, and culture. In doing so, they try to distinguish themselves from other settings. But what is happening is that they are creating a uniqueness paradox, claiming uniqueness when they are, in fact, not unique (Martin, Feldman, Hatch, Sitkin, 1983).

This study illustrated how both sites believe they are unique and distinct from other healthcare settings. But claiming to be unique creates more tension for providers. Most of the practices that are considered unique have become institutionalized, thereby making whatever was considered unique, routine. For example, in the hospice, one of the unique qualities is the hospitality cart that comes around every afternoon at 4pm offering patients and their visitors a beverage and snack. Patients and families frequently ask when the hospitality cart will arrive. They wait for it and many patients even structure their afternoon around the "unique" hospitality cart because it made them feel like they were at home having a choice over what to drink and eat. But the "unique" hospitality cart became inherently standardized, routine, and organized. The hospitality cart lost its uniqueness as a consequence of becoming an institutionalized practice. Even more, it created a tension around patients desiring the cart every day at 4pm but also a disdain for something not routine in an environment built around so many routines and protocols.

Understanding the uniqueness paradox helps us see further that practices of handling death are not unique either. More, it has helped underscore that death is not a uniform event whose meanings are universal and accessible to everyone, but it is an event that wants to be unique and different from something else. Further, uniqueness sets boundaries around understanding individuals and the work they do.

Uniqueness helps providers organize their experience. "We are different from a hospital setting and won't try to keep you alive on unnecessary machines." "Or, we won't stop caring for you like they stop doing at hospice." The uniqueness paradox has a way of mystifying all things. Specifically, the uniqueness paradox in many ways often prevents us from asking questions when someone tells us they work at hospice or the ED. "Ohhhh, I can't imagine," becomes a consistent response that unfortunately closes communication and prevents a discussion from taking place. But this is the very moment we need to start talking in an effort to understand the world as they experience it in the name of caring for and healing our many ailments. This book has shown how much these practitioners enjoy talking about their work and underscored how they also need to be cared for, engaged with, and listened to as our healthcare system seeks reformation.

This book, like all books, has limitations. Specifically, I chose to work through the challenges of representation by using alternative forms of writing such as autoethnography and narrative. This decision, in part, allowed me to escape the constraints of traditional writing as well as lessen the dangers of speaking for others. I realize, however, that in taking this decision to incorporate alternative forms of writing I might potentially make the reader feel uncomfortable who may be more sensitive to these types of writing or take these pages as less serious. The goal is just the opposite. Further, I am also aware that like any form of writing, choosing a new form of expression can simultaneously inhibit other forms.

Another limitation of this book is that in trying to provide a descriptive and honest account of the messiness of healthcare, this analysis is not theoretically rich or rigorous. Further, this study does a better job of raising questions than of answering questions from a theoretical perspective. Another limitation of the study is the enormous ethical commitments it has demanded of me. As a result, I got caught between staying in and leaving these settings, and I left them both feeling exhausted, frustrated, and vulnerable. This in turn made me take a break from this study to literally heal before writing the report. The other limitations of this study I will address by outlining directions for future research.

First, I think a substantive understanding of the ED and the hospice can be incorporated into medical training and teaching so that providers may begin talking about the real difficulty of this work. If instructors so desire, we may begin to incorporate systems and practices that help to heal the healers and their own personal relationships and struggles. Even more, future research into medical education should explore how a more fragmented understanding of clinical life can generate better models of communication and decision making that can respond to the changing health care environment using models and culture beyond the U.S. borders.

Second, future research in end-of-life discourse should examine the role of emotional labor and burnout. If I were to continue with this project, I would carefully focus on how discourses expose the consequences of emotional labor and potential burnout for making meaningful choices around the end of life. Third, future research should incorporate the importance of palliative care. Although I used the term sparingly in this study, I used the philosophy. Future research should expand understandings of palliative care beyond a distinct form of care delivered by a special team during difficult moments in the trajectory of an illness. Palliate literally means to make better. Therefore, every one of the providers on these pages endlessly palliated others, just under different guises. That said, I encourage this research area to explore how providers palliate others and each other and how more providers can do so instead of isolating it as a "specialty" or "emphasis" in medical care and medical education.

Finally, future research should seek to expand our thinking of identity and identification in light of more stigmatized work with institutions that often act like "total institutions" and where work always stays with you, even when providers leave the ED and the hospice to go home (Goffman, 1961; Goffman, 1963; Tompkins & Cheney, 1983). The future research agenda is large and so, too, should be our motivation for exploring the intersections of organizational and health communication.

Moreover, I would encourage scholars to continue offering new insights regarding the storied nature of organizational and clinical life. Both organizational and clinical life is communicated and narrated through stories, because stories are essential to communicating about and organizing health. Paying greater attention to these stories not only offers frameworks for interpreting how health is constituted, but also takes us beyond the realm of the biomedical to the human dimensions of individual health and healing. Further, "stories can heal and they can offer new ways of imagining how the interstices of the mind, body, and spirit rupture our ontological and epistemological foundations and create new openings" (Zoller & Dutta, 2008, p. 462). In short, we can augment dominant ways of knowing through stories and our other senses.

Stories, however, were not my only access to understanding these places. What mattered most was being there to feel lived experience unfold and to be part of these interactions. For these were the moments I understood the most. Together, I hope these stories, voices, and experiences have colored an important picture of the intricate rhythms of these places that are organizing meanings about death as well as helping to re-organize the challenges and opportunities of coordinating care around the end of life.

Closing

The ED and hospice communicate comfort and discomfort. They embrace courage in the name of fear. They are filled with compassion. They are full of incredible knowledge. They are places that surprise, disappoint, and scare me. They make me feel free and imprisoned. They are places people come to for help and hope. And they provide immediate and prolonged answers to those who come close. But above all, they are places that beat, bleed, and breathe meanings surrounding the sacredness and fragility of life and death into all those who come near. Through my own engagement, these places have essentially provided their own rhythm for understanding care at the end of life that is part artistic and part improvisation.

In closing, if this book has challenged your understanding of clinical life to be something other than "normal," and "non-messy," I am happy. And if the narratives that have been slivered into this project in much the same way that they have slivered into my heart and train of thought as I write, have somehow slivered a piece of your heart, my goals have been met.

For if nothing else, my hope is for you, the patient, to contemplate the accounts and stories from providers at both sites to understand their own experiences, fears, frustrations, demands, expectations, and energies that they intricately balance when you are in their presence next.

My hope is for you, the provider, to gain a better understanding and appreciation for the tightrope you all endlessly walk when caring for others. And in listening to other providers, I hope you have questioned some of your very own practices as well as wonder what it would look like, feel like, and sound like to start doing things a little differently in your practice.

And my hope for you, the researcher, is to have become a little more willing to lay yourself bare when you write, think, feel, and inquire. For if nothing else, I hope you are motivated to underscore how our very own discourses can be oppressive, confusing, and closed for many who do not speak this language. Further, I challenge you to "let yourself go" a little so as to have your voice and work be more accessible to audiences other than your own, and to be vulnerable to some of the challenges and failures of our work so that others may learn from them, and with you.

Finally, my hope for us all is to listen to the voices on these pages to understand the consequences of care-giving and the need to make caring for each other, and ourselves, a common facet of life. Even more, I hope these pages have generated small and large discussions where none seemed needed before. Care, one of the most deeply shared feelings on earth, has become one of the most expensive human practices. But care is a universal need that everyone benefits from at some point in their life, whether in public or private. We are at a crisis surrounding the meanings of health care in general and death in particular. Together, these stories and perspectives paint one suggestion into the crisis over meaning and some of the issues and tensions individuals and caregivers face while arguing that well care for individuals, especially aging individuals, is fundamental to creating a developed, ethical, and engaged society.

Health care will continue to change. And we will continue to live longer, treat and suffer from more complicated and long-term diseases, coordinate decisions with more people than ever before, and rather than call it a provider "shortage," creatively think of ways to better allocate resources and providers' time, pay, and responsibilities. Therefore, we all must keep up with medical changes and enact a vocabulary and ethics that are responsive to the changing nature of talking about and making decisions surrounding the end of life with those we love, and those that love us. Because if not us, then who?

REFERENCES

Alcott, L. (1991–1992). The problem of speaking for others. *Cultural Critique*, Winter, 5–32.

Alvesson, M., & Deetz, S. (2000). *Doing critical management research*. London: Sage.

Alvesson, M., & Deetz, S. (1996). Critical theory and postmodern approaches to organizational studies. In S. R. Clegg, C. Hardy, & W. R. Nord (Eds.), *Handbook of organization studies* (pp. 191–217). Thousand Oaks, CA: Sage.

American College of Emergency Physicians. Report from a Roundtable discussion: Meeting the challenge of emergency department overcrowding/boarding. American College of Emergency Physicians. http://www.emra.org

American Hospital Association (1974–2002). http://www.aha.org/about/index.shtml

Armstrong, D. (2003). *Outline of sociology as applied to medicine* (5th Ed.). Oxford, UK: Oxford University Press.

Armstrong, D. (2002). *A new history of identity: A sociology of medical knowledge*. Basingstoke: Palgrave.

Arney, W. R., & Bergen, B. J. (1984). *Medicine and the management of living: Taming the last great beast*. Chicago, IL: University of Chicago Press.

Atkinson, P. (1995). *Medical talk and medical work: The liturgy of the clinic*. London: Sage.

Babrow, A. S., & Mattson, M. (2003). Theorizing about health communication. In T. L. Thompson, A. M. Dorsey, K. I. Miller, & R. Parrott (Eds.), *Handbook of health communication* (pp. 35–61). Mahwah, NJ: Erlbaum.

Baer, H., Singer, M., & Johnsen, J. (1986). Toward a critical medical anthropology. *Social Science and Medicine*, 23, 95–98.

Becker, E. (1997). *The denial of death*. New York: Free Press.

Berger, P. L., & Luckmann, T. (1966). *The social construction of reality: A treatise in the sociology of knowledge*. Garden City, NY: Doubleday.

Bern-Klug, M., & Chapin, R. (1999). The changing demography of death in the United States: Implications for human service workers. In B. de Vries (ed.), *End of life issues: Interdisciplinary and multidimensional perspectives*. New York: Springer.

Bradshaw, A. (1996). Recovering the tradition of patient-centered nursing. In Fulford, B., Ersser, S. & Hope, T. (eds.) *Essential practice in patient-centered care*. Oxford: Blackwell Science.

Broadfoot, K. J. (2003). *Disarming genes and the discursive reorganizing of knowledge, technology and self in medicine*. Unpublished doctoral dissertation. University of Colorado, Boulder.

Broadfoot, K. J. (2005). "She's come undone!": Engaging scholarship and viral research. In J. L. Simpson & P. Shockley-Zalabak (Eds.), *Engaging communication, transforming organizations: Scholarship of engagement in action* (pp. 98–112). Cresskill, NJ: Hampton Press.

Browning, L. (1992). Lists and stories in organizational communication. *Communication Theory, 2*, 281–302.

Buber, M. (1958). *I and thou*. New York: Charles Scribner's Sons.

Buber, M. (1973). *Meetings*. LaSalle, IL: Open Court Publishing Company.

Burawoy, M. (1991). *Ethnography unbound: Power and resistance in the modern metropolis*. Berkeley, CA: University of California Press.

Callahan, D. (2000). *The troubled dream of life: In search of a peaceful death*. New York: Touchstone Books.

Cassell, E. J. (2004). *The nature of suffering and the goals of medicine* (2nd ed.) New York: Oxford University Press.

Centers for Disease Control and Prevention (2009). The Power of Prevention: Chronic disease…the public health challenge of the 21st century. http://www.cdc.gov/chronicdisease/pdf/2009-power-of-prevention.pdf

Centers for Disease Control and Prevention (2012). Centers for Disease Control and Prevention Fact Sheet. http://www.cdc.gov

Centers for Disease Control and Prevention (2013). *The State of Aging and Health in America 2013*. Atlanta, GA: Centers for Disease Control and Prevention, US Dept of Health and Human Services. http://www.cdc.gov/features/agingandhealth/state_of_aging_and_health_in_america_2013.pdf

Centers for Medicare and Medicaid Services (2010), *Medicare Spending Fact Sheet*, http://cms.hhs.gov

Charmaz, K. (1980). *The social reality of death: Death in contemporary America*. Reading, MA: Addison-Wesley Publishing.

Charon, R. (2006). *Narrative medicine: Honoring the stories of illness*. New York: Oxford University Press.

Chittenden, E. H., Clark, S. T., & Pantilat, S. Z. (2006). Discussing resuscitation preferences with patients: Challenges and rewards. *Journal of Hospital Medicine, 4*, 231–240.

Clair, R. (2003). *Expressions of ethnography: Novel approaches to qualitative methods*. Albany: SUNY Press.

Clair, R. (1998). *Organizing silence: A world of possibilities*. Albany: State University of New York Press.

Clifford, J., & Marcus, G. (1986). *Writing culture: The poetics and politics of ethnography*. Berkeley, CA: University of California Press.

Congressional Budget Office (1999). Retrieved May 2009: http://www.cbo.gov/publications/bysubject.cfm?cat=35

Conquergood, D. (1991). Rethinking ethnography: Towards a critical cultural politics. *Communication Monographs, 58*, 179–194.

Corr, C. A. (1997). *Death and dying: Life and living*. Belmont, CA: Wadsworth.

The Dartmouth Atlas of Health Care on End of Life Care, 2010. http://www.dartmouthatlas.org/keyissues/issue.aspx?con=2944

Deetz, S. (2001). Conceptual foundations for organizational communication studies. In F. M. Jablin & L. L. Putnam (Eds.), *The new handbook of organizational communication: Advances in theory, research, and methods* (pp. 2–46). Thousand Oaks, CA: Sage.

Deetz, S. (1992). *Democracy in an age of corporate colonization: Developments in communication and the politics of everyday life*. Albany, NY: SUNY Press.

Deetz, S., & Mumby, D. (1985). Metaphors, information, and power. In B. Ruben (Ed.), *Information and Behavior, Volume 1*, (pp. 369–386). New Brunswick, NJ: Transaction Press.

Deetz, S., & Radford, G. (2008). *Communication theory at the crossroads: Responding to globalization, pluralism and collaborative needs*. Oxford: Blackwell Publications.

Denzin, N. K. (1991). Representing lived experiences in ethnographic texts. *Studies in Symbolic Interaction, 15*, 59–70.

Denzin, N. K. (1997). *Interpretive ethnography: Ethnographic practices for the 21ˢᵗ century*. Thousand Oaks, CA: Sage.

Denzin, N. K. (2003). The art and politics of interpretation. In N. Denzin & Y. Lincoln (Eds.), *Collecting and interpreting qualitative materials*. Thousand Oaks, CA: Sage.

Department of Health and Human Services Centers for Medicare & Medicaid Services. Medicare Learning Network Payment System Fact Sheet Series, December 2013.

Eisenberg, E. M. (1990). Jamming: Transcendence through organizing. *Communication Research, 17*, 139–164.

Eisenberg, E., Murphy, K., Wears, R., Schenkel, S., Perry, S., & Vanderhoef, M. (2005). Communication in emergency medicine: Implications for patient safety. *Communication Monographs, 72*, 390–413.

Ellingson, L. L. (2005). *Communicating in the clinic: Negotiating frontstage and backstage teamwork*. Cresskill, NJ: Hampton Press.

Ellingson, L. L. (1998). "Then you know how I feel": Empathy, identification, and reflexivity in fieldwork. *Qualitative Inquiry, 4*, 492–514.

Fairhurst, G. T., & Putnam, L. L. (2004). Organizations as discursive constructions. *Communication Theory, 14*, 5–26.

Foster, E. (2007). *Communicating at the end of life: Finding magic in the mundane*. Mahwah, NJ: Lawrence Erlbaum Associates.

Foucault, M. (1973). *The birth of the clinic: An archaeology of medical perception*. New York: Pantheon Books.

Foucault, M. (1976). *The history of sexuality: Vol. 1.* New York: Pantheon.

Foucault, M. (1979). *The history of sexuality: Introduction.* London: Allen Lane.

Frank, A. (1995). *The wounded storyteller: Body, illness, and ethics.* Chicago: University of Chicago Press.

Gawande, A. (2009). The cost conundrum: Expensive health care can be harmful. *The New Yorker* (June1).

Geertz, C. (1973). *The interpretation of cultures.* New York: Basic Books.

Gergen, M. M., & Gergen, K. J. (2002). Ethnographic representation as relationship. In Bochner & Ellis (Eds.), *Ethnographically speaking: Autoethnography, literature and aesthetics* (pp. 11–33). Walnut Creek, CA: Alta Mira Press.

Giddens, A. (1979). *Central problems in social theory.* Berkeley: University of California Press.

Giddens, A. (1984). *The constitution of society.* Berkeley: University of California Press.

Giddens, A. (1991). *Modernity and self-identity: Self and society in the late modern age.* Stanford, CA: Stanford University Press.

Goffman, E. (1989). On fieldwork. *Journal of Contemporary Ethnography, 18,* 123–132.

Goffman, E. (1963). *Stigma: Notes on the management of spoiled identity.* New York: Simon & Schuster.

Goffman, E. (1961). *Asylums: Essays on the social situation of mental patients and other inmates.* New York: Doubleday.

González, M. C. (2003). An ethics for post-colonial ethnography. In R. Clair (Ed.). *Expressions of ethnography.* Albany, NY: SUNY Press.

González, M. C. (2000). The four seasons of ethnography: A creation-centered ontology for ethnography. *International Journal of Intercultural Relations, 24,* 623–650.

Goodman, J. C., Villareal, P., & Jones, B. (2010). The social cost of adverse medical events, and what we can do about it. *Health Affairs, 30*(4), 590–595. doi: 10.1377/hlthaff.2010.1256

Groopman, J. (2007). *How doctors think.* New York: Houghton Mifflin Company.

Han, P. K. J., Keranen, L. B., Lescisin, D. A., & Arnold, R. M. (2005). The palliative care clinical evaluation exercise (CEX): An experience-based intervention for teaching end-of-life communication skills. *Academic Medicine, 80,* 669–676.

Hawes, L. (1974). Social collectivities as communication: Perspective on organizational behavior. *Quarterly Journal of Speech, 60,* 497–502.

Hickman, S. E. (2002). Improving communication near the end of life. *American Behavioral Scientist, 46,* 252–267.

Hirschmann, K. (1999). Blood, vomit, and communication: The days and nights of an intern on call. *Health Communication, 11,* 35–57.

Hunter, K. M. (1991). *Doctors' stories: The narrative structure of medical knowledge.* Princeton, NJ: Princeton University Press.

Illich, I. (1976). *Limits to medicine: Medical nemesis, the exploration of health.* London: Marion Boyars.

Irwin, H. (1989). Health communication: The research agenda. *Media Information Australia, 54,* 32–40.

Keaton, B. F. (2007). Emergency medicine: A national perspective. In K. E. Harkin & J. T. Cuchman (Eds.), *Medical student survival guide*, *2nd edition* (pp. 5–6). Irving, TX: Emergency Medicine Residents' Association.

Keranen, L. (2007). "Cause someday we all must die": Rhetoric, agency and the case of the "patient" preferences worksheet. *Quarterly Journal of Speech, 93*, 179–211.

Kreps, G. L. (1989). Setting the agenda for health communication research and development: Scholarship that can make a difference. *Health Communication, 1*, 11–15.

Littlewood, J. (1993). The denial of death and rites of passage in contemporary societies. In D. Clark (Ed.), *The sociology of death: Theory, culture, practice*. Cambridge, MA: Blackwell.

Lupton, D. (2003). *Medicine as culture* (2nd ed.). London: Sage.

Lupton, D. (1994). Toward the development of critical health communication praxis. *Health Communication, 6*, 55–67.

Lynn, J. (2004). *Sick to death and not going to take it anymore!: Reforming health care for the last years of life*. Berkeley: University of California Press.

Martin, J. (1990). Deconstructing organizational taboos: The suppression of gender conflict in organizations. *Organization science, 1*, 339–359.

Martin, J., Feldman, M. S., Hatch, M. J., & Sitkin, S. B. (1983). The uniqueness paradox in organizational stories. *Administrative Science Quarterly, 28*(3), 438–453.

Mies, M. (1983). Toward a methodology for feminist research. In G. Bowles & R. Duelli Klein (Eds.), *Theories of women's studies*. Boston: Routledge & Kegan Paul.

Miller, G. (1994). Towards ethnographies of institutional discourse: Prospects and suggestions. *Journal of Contemporary Ethnography, 23*, 280–306.

Mishler, E. G. (1984). *The discourse of medicine: Dialectic of medical interviews*. Norwood, NJ: Ablex Publishing.

Mokros, H. B., & Deetz, S. (1996). What counts as real?: A constitutive view of communication and the disenfranchised in the context of health. In E. B. Ray (Ed.), *Communication and disenfranchisement: Social health issues and implications* (pp. 29–44). Mahwah, NJ: Lawrence Erlbaum.

Morrison, S. R., Penrod, J. D, Cassel, B. J., Caust-Ellenbogen, M., Litke, A., Spragens, L., & Meier, D. E. (2008). Cost savings associated with US hospital palliative care consultation programs. *Arch Internal Medicine, 168*(16): 1783–1790.

National Council for Palliative Care. Retrieved May 2009: www.ncpc.org.uk

National Hospice and Palliative Care Organization, Retrieved May 2009: http://www.nhpco.org

Pagis, M. (2010) Producing intersubjectivity in silence: An ethnography of meditation practices." *Ethnography* 11: 309–328.

Picard, M. (1952). *The world of silence* (S. Godman, Trans.). South Bend, IN: Regnery/Gateway. (Original work published 1948).

Ragan, S. L., Wittenberg-Lyles, E. M., Goldsmith, J., & Sanchez-Reilly, S. (2008). *Communication as comfort: Multiple voices in palliative care*. New York: Routledge.

Rose, N. (1994). Medicine, history and the present. In C. Jones & R. Porter (Eds.), *Reassessing Foucault: Power, medicine and the body* (pp. 48–71). London: Routledge.

Rose, N. (2002). *Governing the soul: The shaping of the private self.* (2nd ed.) London: Free Association Books.

Saunders, C. (1967). *The management of terminal illness.* London: Hospital Medicine Publications.

Saunders, C. (2003). A voice for the voiceless. In B. Monroe & D. Oliviere (Eds.), *Patient participation in palliative care: A voice for the voiceless.* Oxford: Oxford University Press.

Schön, D. A. (1983). *The reflective practitioner: How professionals think in action.* New York: Basic Books.

Seale, C. (1998). *Constructing death: The sociology of dying and bereavement.* Cambridge, UK: Cambridge University Press.

Segal, J. Z. (2005). *Health and the rhetoric of medicine.* Carbondale: Southern Illinois University Press.

Sellers, S. C., & Haag, B. A. (1998). Spiritual nursing interventions. *Journal of Holistic Nursing, 16,* 338–354.

Street, R. L., Jr. (2003). Communication in medical encounters: An ecological perspective. In T. Thompson, A. Dorsey, K. Miller, & R. Parrott (eds.), *The handbook of health communication* (pp. 63–89). Mahwah, NJ: Erlbaum.

SUPPORT Investigators (1995). A controlled trial to improve care for seriously ill, hospitalized patients: The Study to Understand Prognoses and Preferences for Outcomes and Treatments (SUPPORT). *Journal of the American Medical Association, 274,* 1591–8.

Taylor, B. C., & Trujillo, N. (2001). Qualitative research methods. In F. M. Jablin & L. L. Putnam (Eds.). *The new handbook of organizational communication: Advances in theory, research, and methods* (pp. 161–193). Thousand Oaks, CA: Sage.

Thackaberry, J. A. (2004). Discursive opening and closing in organizational self study: Culture as the culprit for safety problems in wildland firefighting. *Management Communication Quarterly, 17,* 319–359.

Tompkins, P. K., & Cheney, G. (1983). Account analysis of organizations: Decision making and identification. In L. Putman & M. Pacanowsky (Eds.), *Communication and organizations: An interpretive approach* (pp. 179–210). Newbury Park, CA: Sage.

Treichler, P. A. (1990). Feminism, medicine, and the meaning of childbirth. In M. Jacobs, E. F. Keller, & S. Shuttleworth (eds.), *Body/Politics: Women and the discourses of science* (pp. 113–138). New York: Routledge.

Ufema, J. (2006). *Insights on death and dying.* Ambler, PA: Lippincott Williams & Wilkins.

Waitzkin, H. (1984). The micropolitics of medicine: a contextual analysis. *International Journal of Health Services, 14,* 339–378.

Wall Street Journal, 2/26/2008 (medicare spending).

Walter, T. (1994). *The revival of death.* East Sussex, UK: Psychology Press..

Watson, T. (2003). Professions and professionalism: Should we jump off the bandwagon, better to study where it is going? *International Studies of Management & Organization, 32,* 93–105.

Weedon, C. (1997). *Feminist practice and poststructuralist theory.* (2nd ed.) Oxford, UK: Blackwell.

Weick, K. (1998). Improvisation as a mindset for organizational analysis. *Organization Science, 9* (5): 543–555.

Wenrich, M. D., Curtis, J. R., Shannon, S. E., Carline, J. D., Ambrozy, D. M., & Ramsey, P. G. (2001). Communication with dying patients within the spectrum of medical care from terminal diagnosis to death. *Archives of Internal Medicine, 161,* 868–874.

West, J. T. (1993). Ethnography and ideology: The politics of cultural representation. *Western Journal of Communication, 57,* 209–220.

Zink. B. J. (2006). *Anyone, anything, anytime: A history of emergency medicine.* Philadelphia, PA: Mosby Elsevier.

Zoller, H. M., & Dutta, M. J. (2008). *Emerging perspectives in health communication: Meaning, culture, and power.* New York: Routledge:

Zoller, H., & Kline, K. (2008). Interpretive and critical contributions to health communication theory. *Communication Yearbook, 32,* 89–135.

INDEX

F

G

H

I

K

L

M

N

O

P

Q

R

S

T

U

V

W

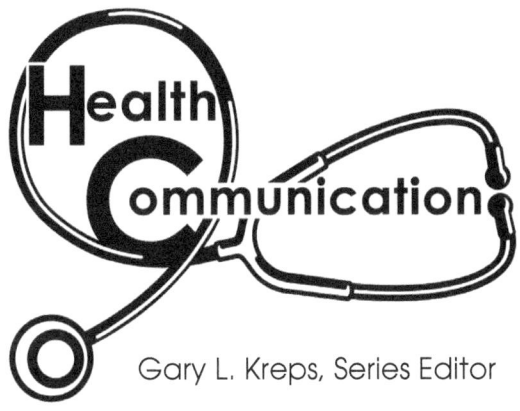

Gary L. Kreps, Series Editor

This series examines the powerful influences of human and mediated communication in delivering care and promoting health.

Books analyze the ways that strategic communication humanizes and increases access to quality care as well as examining the use of communication to encourage proactive health promotion. The books describe strategies for addressing major health issues, such as reducing health disparities, minimizing health risks, responding to health crises, encouraging early detection and care, facilitating informed health decisionmaking, promoting coordination within and across health teams, overcoming health literacy challenges, designing responsive health information technologies, and delivering sensitive end-of-life care.

All books in the series are grounded in broad evidence-based scholarship and are vivid, compelling, and accessible to broad audiences of scholars, students, professionals, and laypersons.

For additional information about this series or for the submission of manuscripts, please contact:

Gary L. Kreps
University Distinguished Professor and Chair, Department of Communication
Director, Center for Health and Risk Communication
George Mason University Science & Technology 2, Suite 230, MS 3D6
Fairfax, VA 22030-4444
gkreps@gmu.edu

To order other books in this series, please contact our Customer Service Department:

(800) 770-LANG (within the U.S.)
(212) 647-7706 (outside the U.S.)
(212) 647-7707 FAX

Or browse online by series:
www.peterlang.com

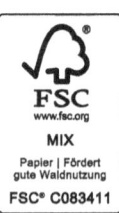

Zeitfracht Medien GmbH
Ferdinand-Jühlke-Straße 7
99095 Erfurt, Deutschland
produktsicherheit@kolibri360.de